AF589570

Children's Advertisement

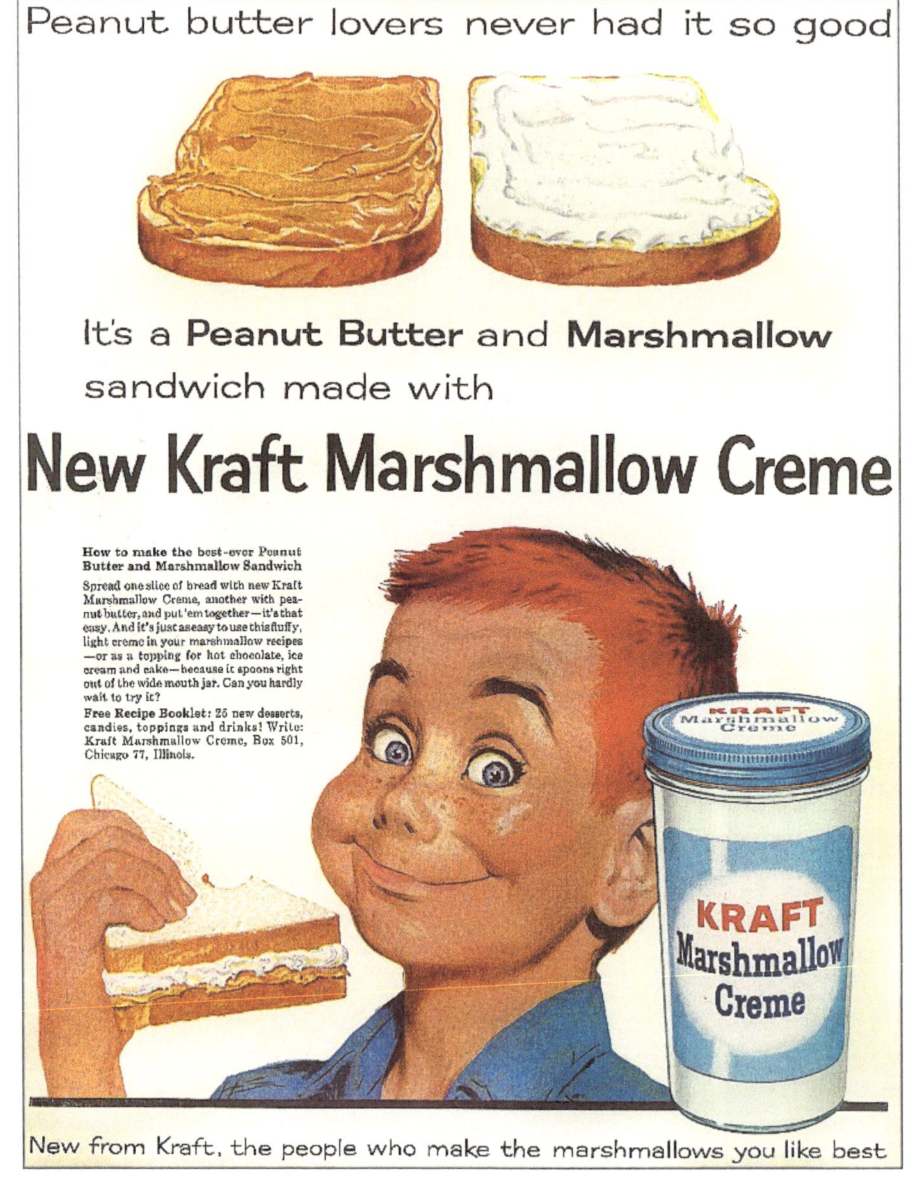

Children's Advertisement

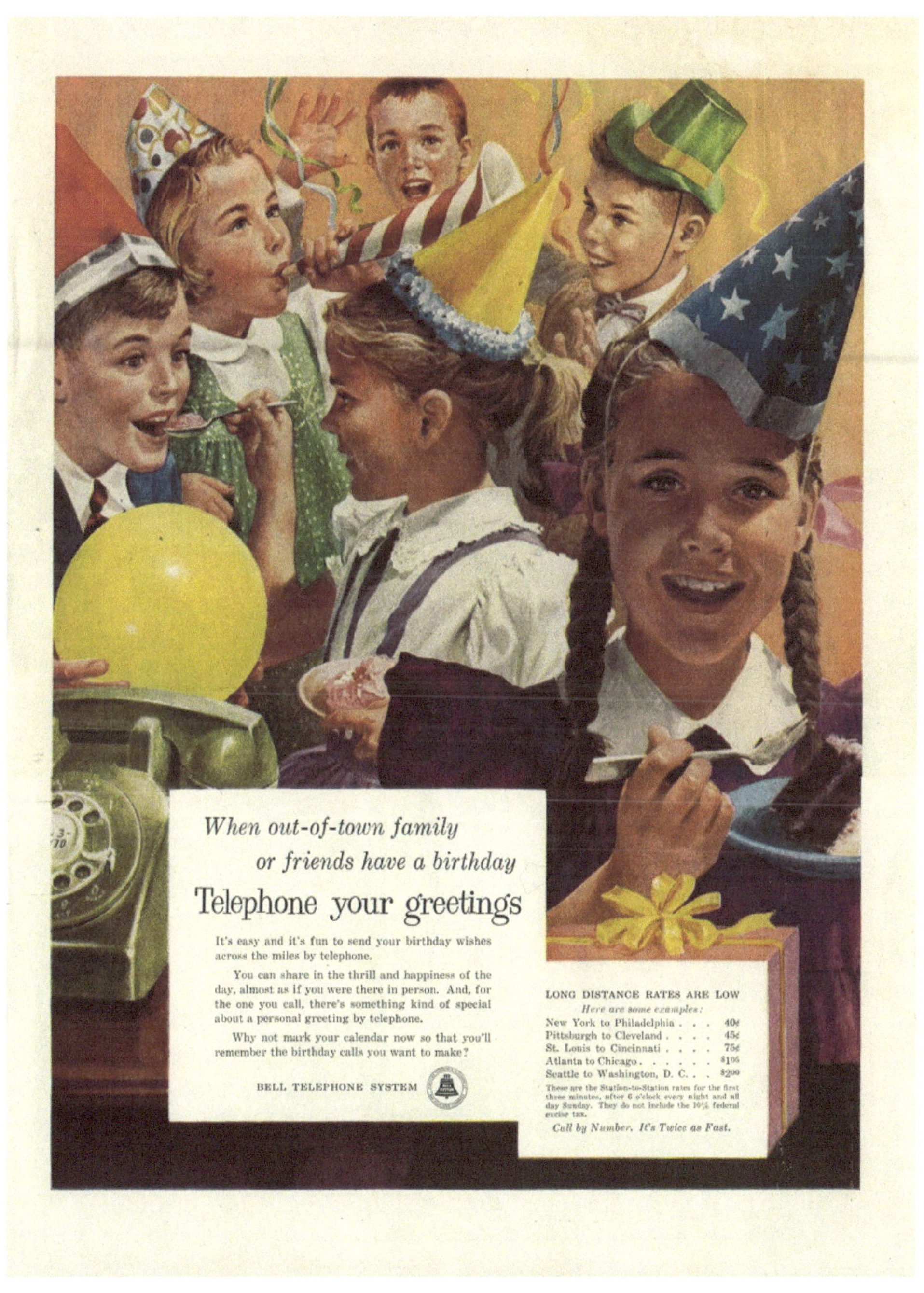

Refreshing Drinks

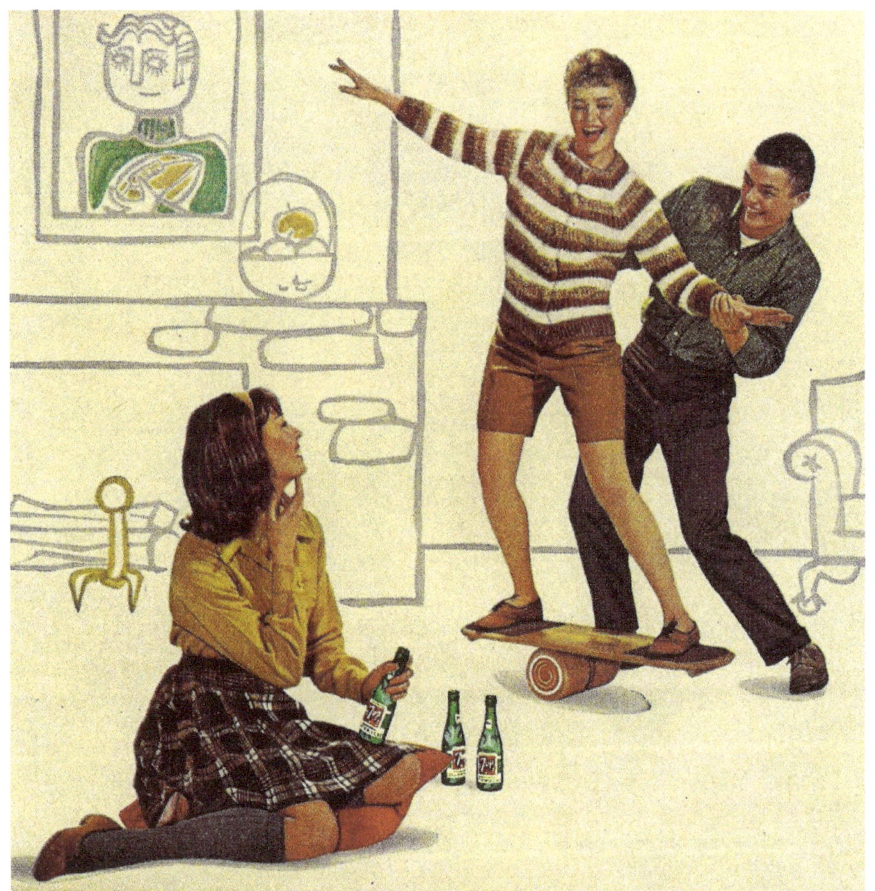

Copyright 1960 by The Seven-Up Company

However you do your rock-and-roll... you'll need the real thirst-quencher!

The faster the action—the thirstier you get—and the more you need 7-Up! With the first sparkling sip, it starts to quench. With the last sparkling sip, thirst is down and out. So when you bring on the fun and games—bring on the 7-Up! It's *always* 7-Up time.

7up

Nothing, nothing, nothing does it like Seven-Up!

Refreshing Drinks

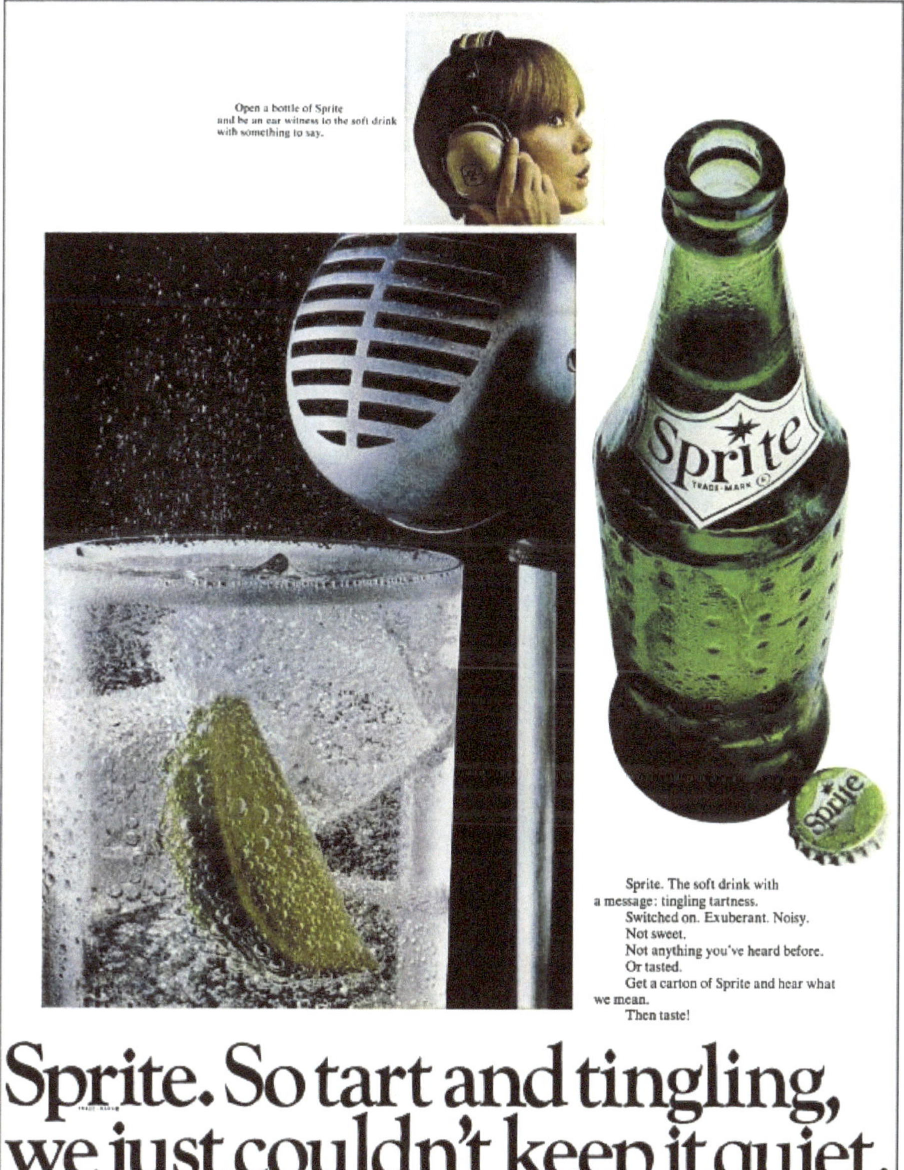

Advertisements for Women

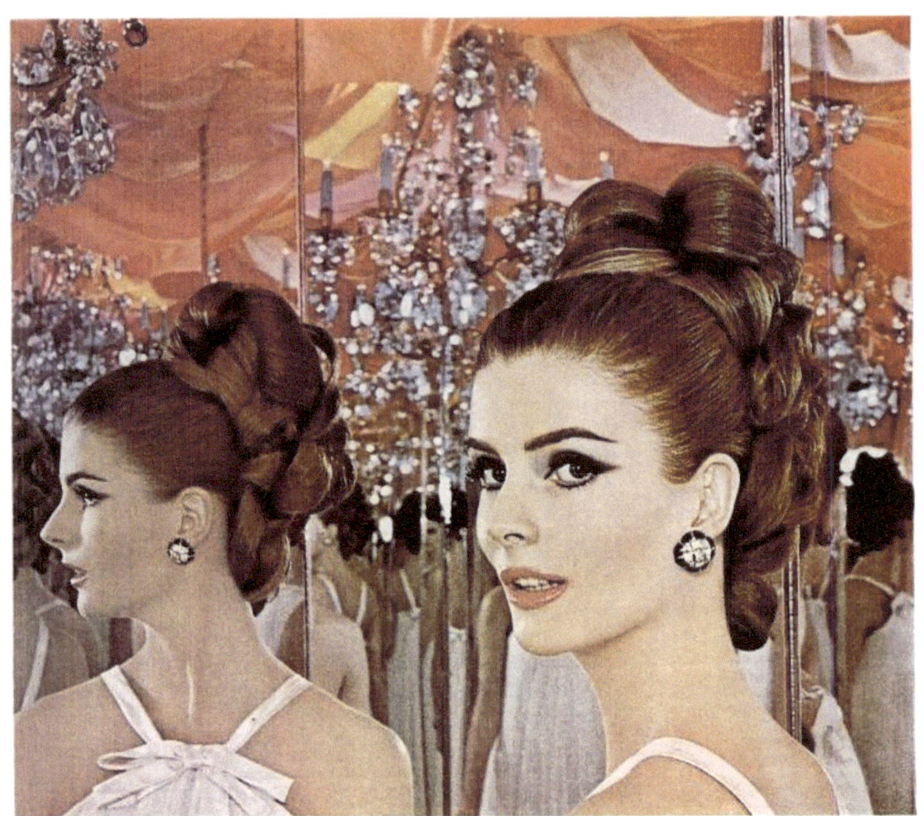

Today's chic is creamy sleek. Why settle for "little-nothing" lips!

MAX FACTOR INTRODUCES
ULTRALUCENT CREME LIPSTICKS

Discovered: a lipstick that knows no dryness— Max Factor's remarkable new UltraLucent Creme. So rich it slithers on like a lick of cream, so dazzling you'd think it was done with mirrors. Max Factor does it with an incredibly creamy new color base that's pure gloss, yet soft and un-greasy! Makes your lips feel different (much yummier). Makes color look different... dewier, *deluged* with glow. In twenty-one colors (eight in a sumptuous new iridescent) that make fashion sit up and purr. Slip into a few. It's like making up with a kiss.

Advertisements for Women

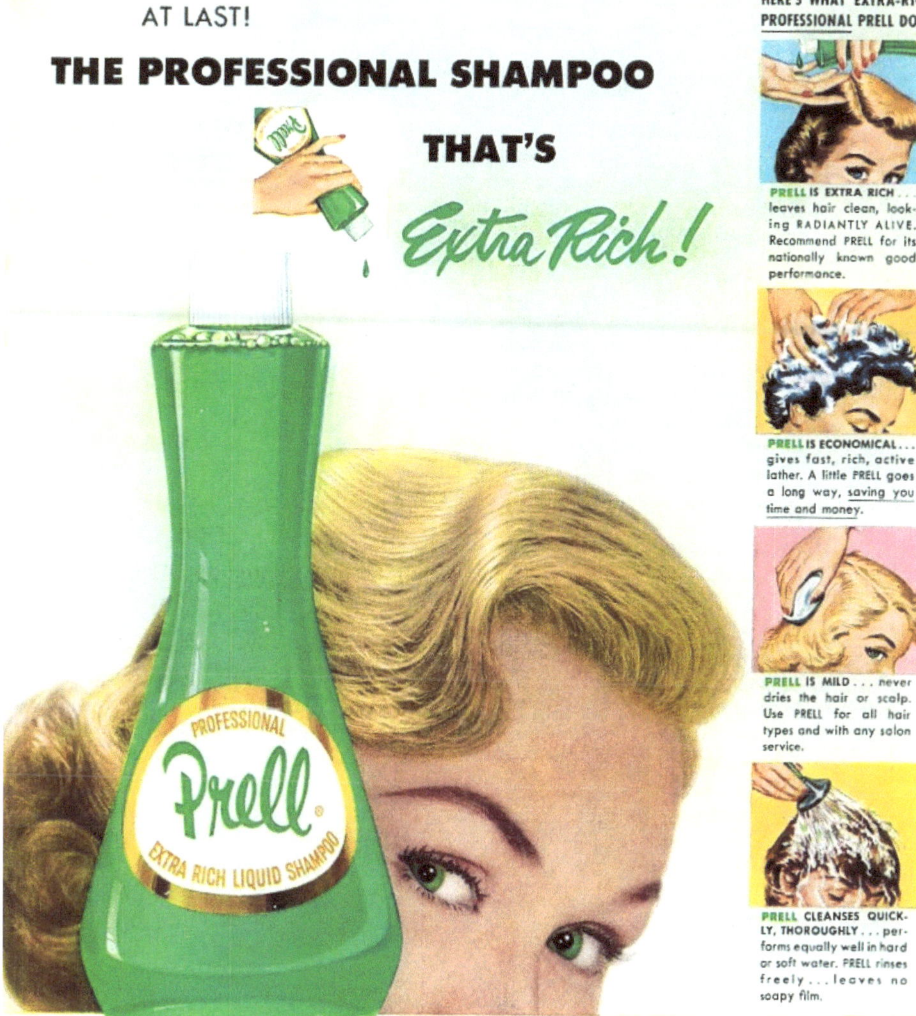

IT'S LIQUID **PRELL** IN A PROFESSIONAL FORMULA AT A COMPETITIVE PRICE!

PRELL—THE PRESTIGE SHAMPOO WOMEN PREFER!

NEW 16 OZ. BOTTLE OF CONCENTRATED LIQUID PRELL MAKES UP INSTANTLY INTO A GALLON OF READY-TO-USE SHAMPOO!

AND: New dispenser cap! Dispenser bottle for your shelves! "Won't-slip" bottle designed to fit your hand!

REGULAR PRICE PER CASE . . . $7.95. SAVE MORE THAN $1.00 WHEN YOU BUY THE 4 BOTTLE CASE $2.25 per bottle in less than case lots.

Best Cars Of The 60s

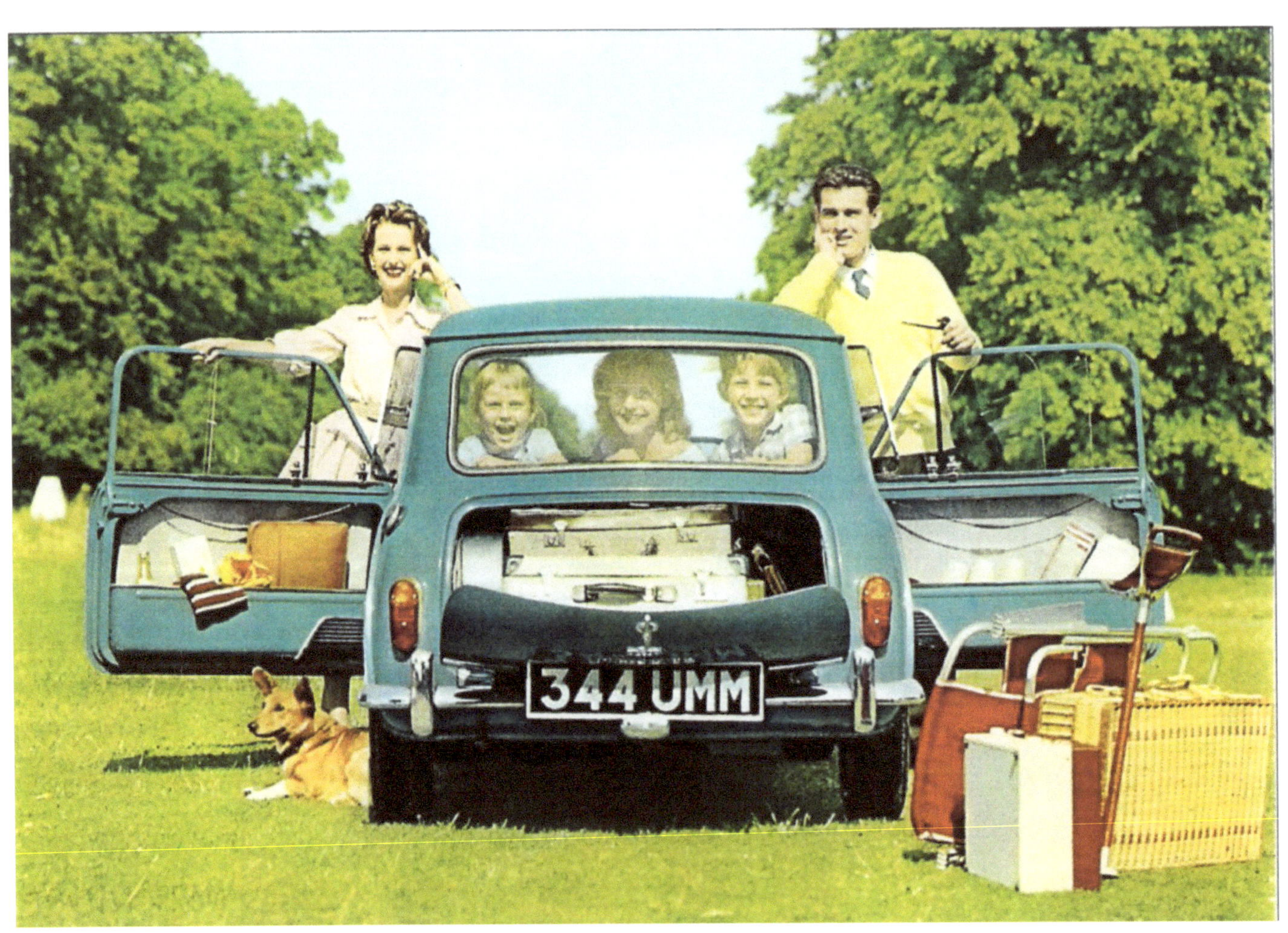

BMC Mini

Best Cars Of The 60s

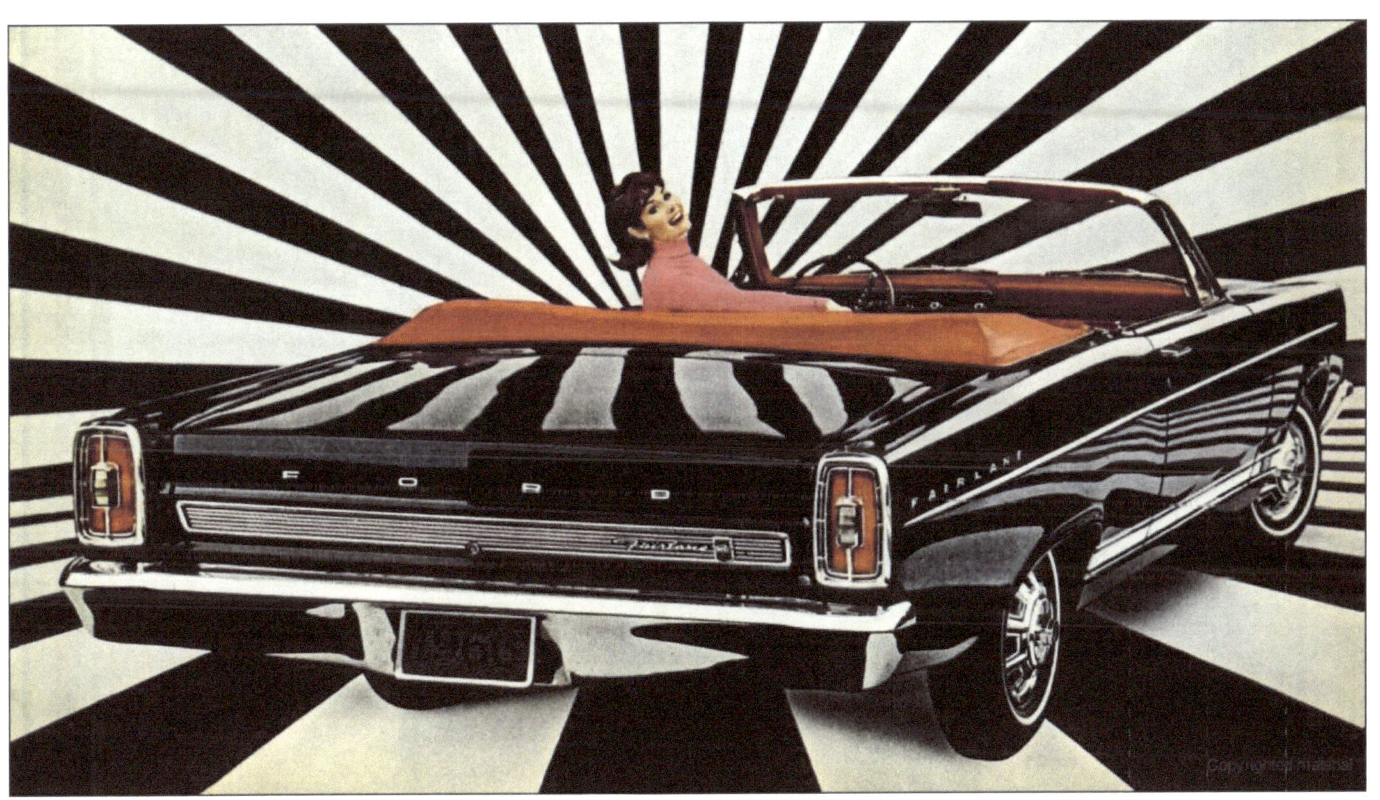

Ford Fairlane

Best Cars Of The 60s

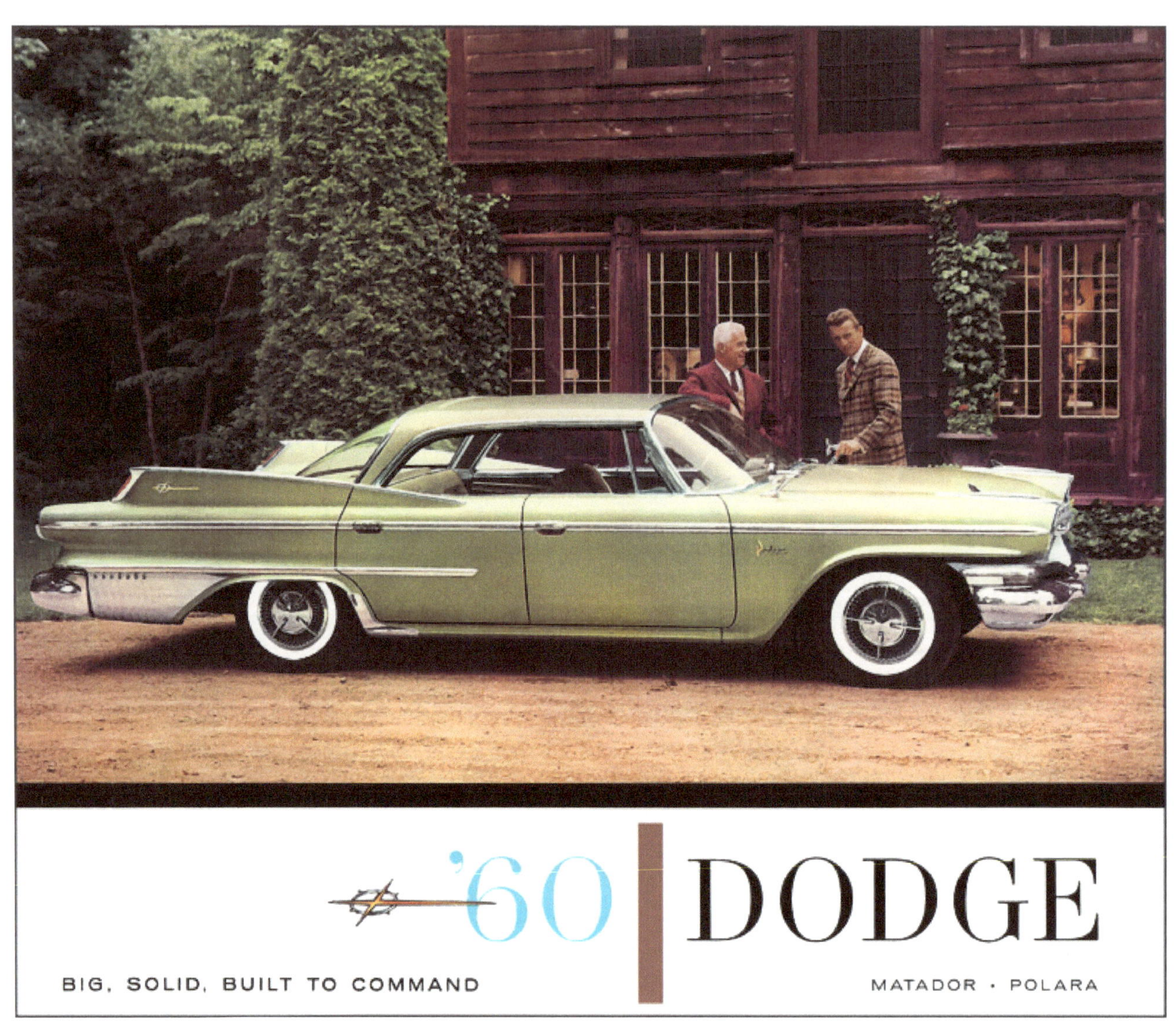

Dodge Polara

Top Actors

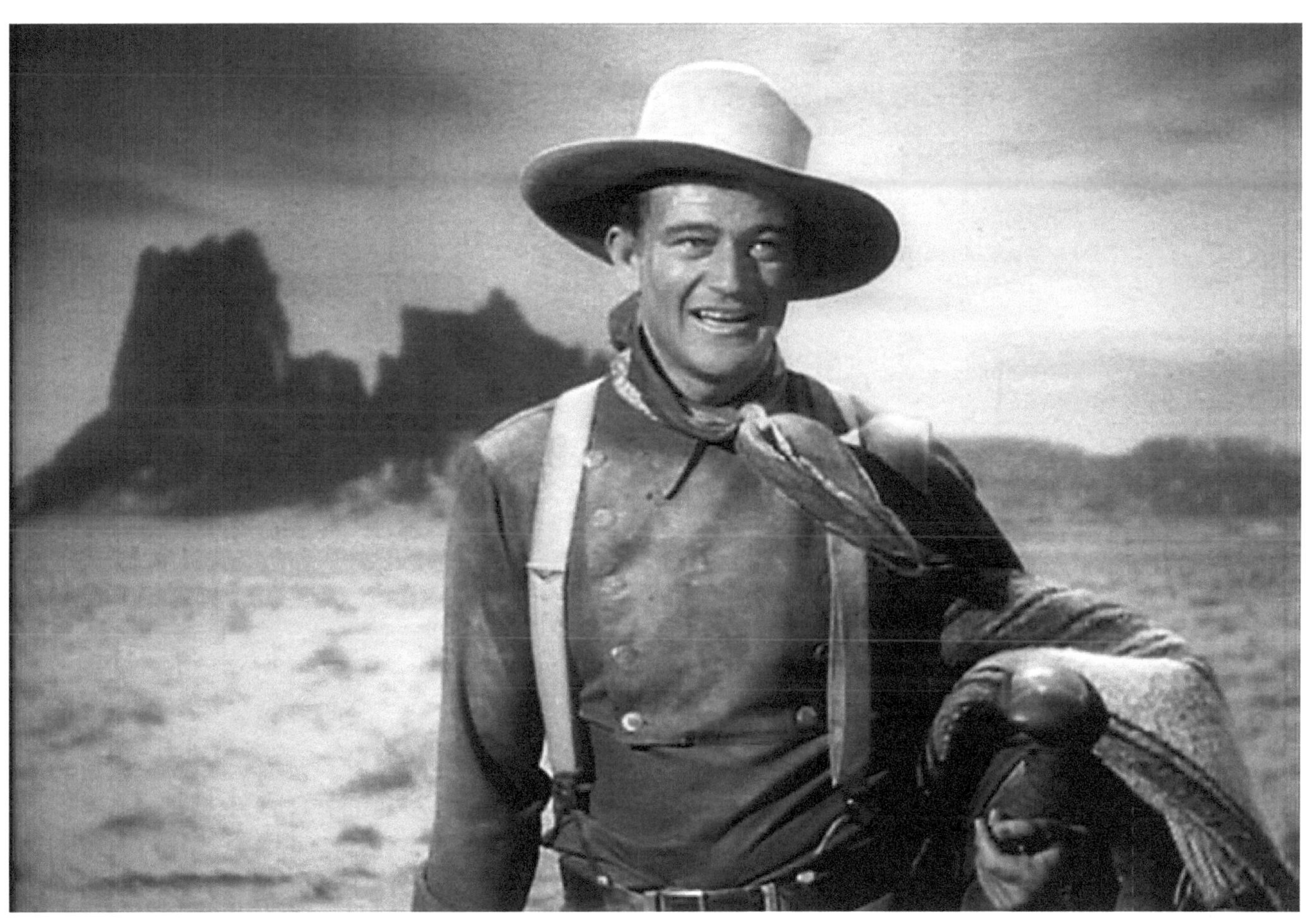

John Wayne

Top Actors

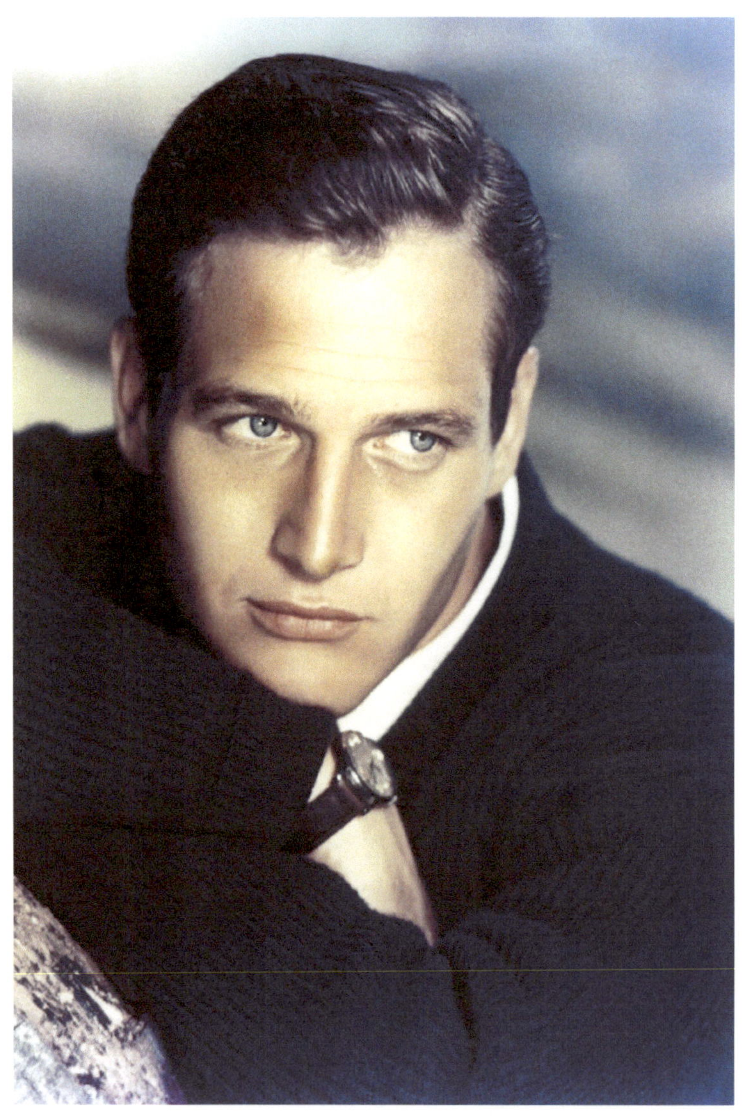

Paul Newman

Top Actresses

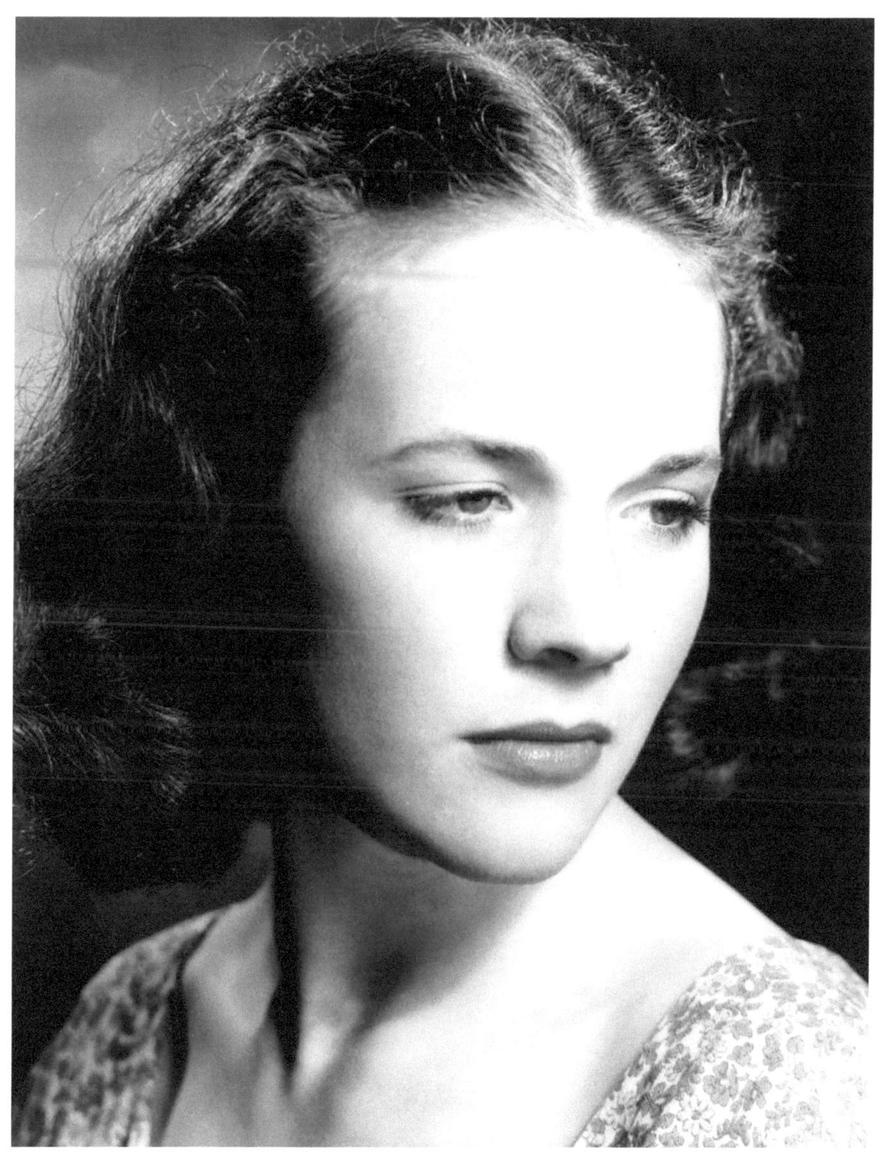

Julie Andrews

Top Actresses

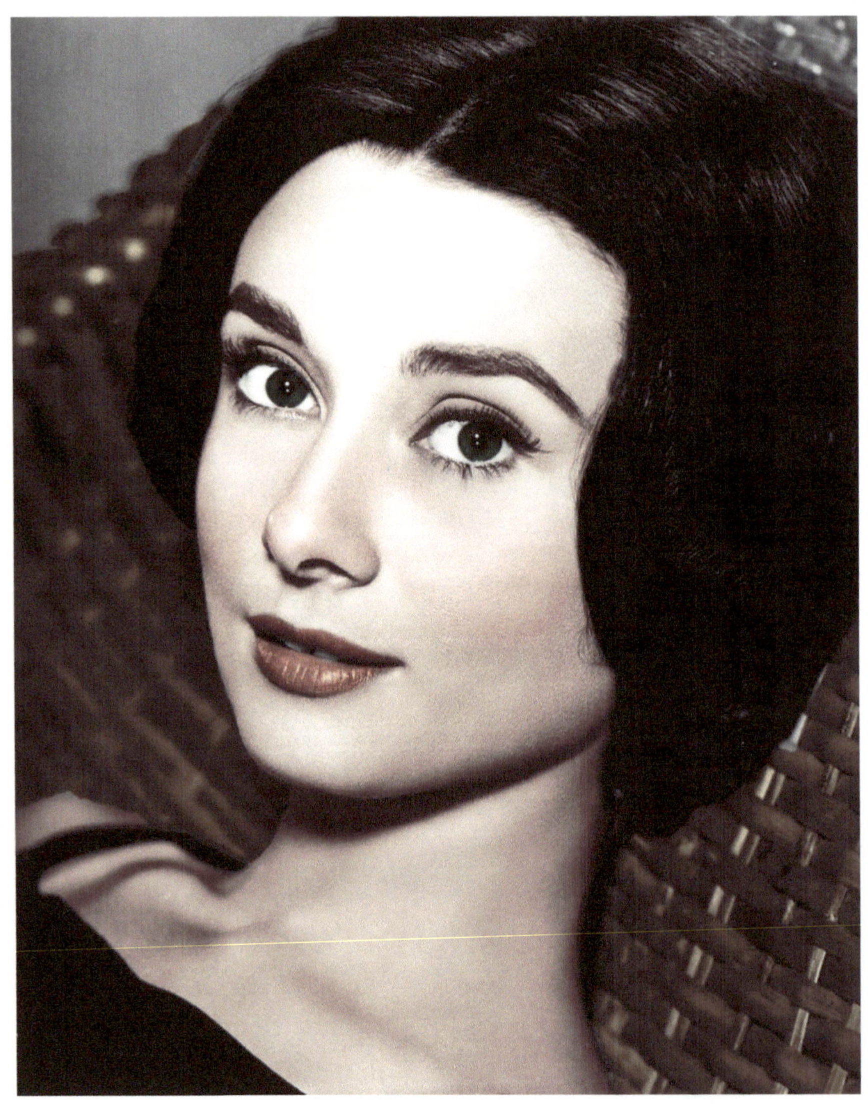

Audrey Hepburn

Famous Icons

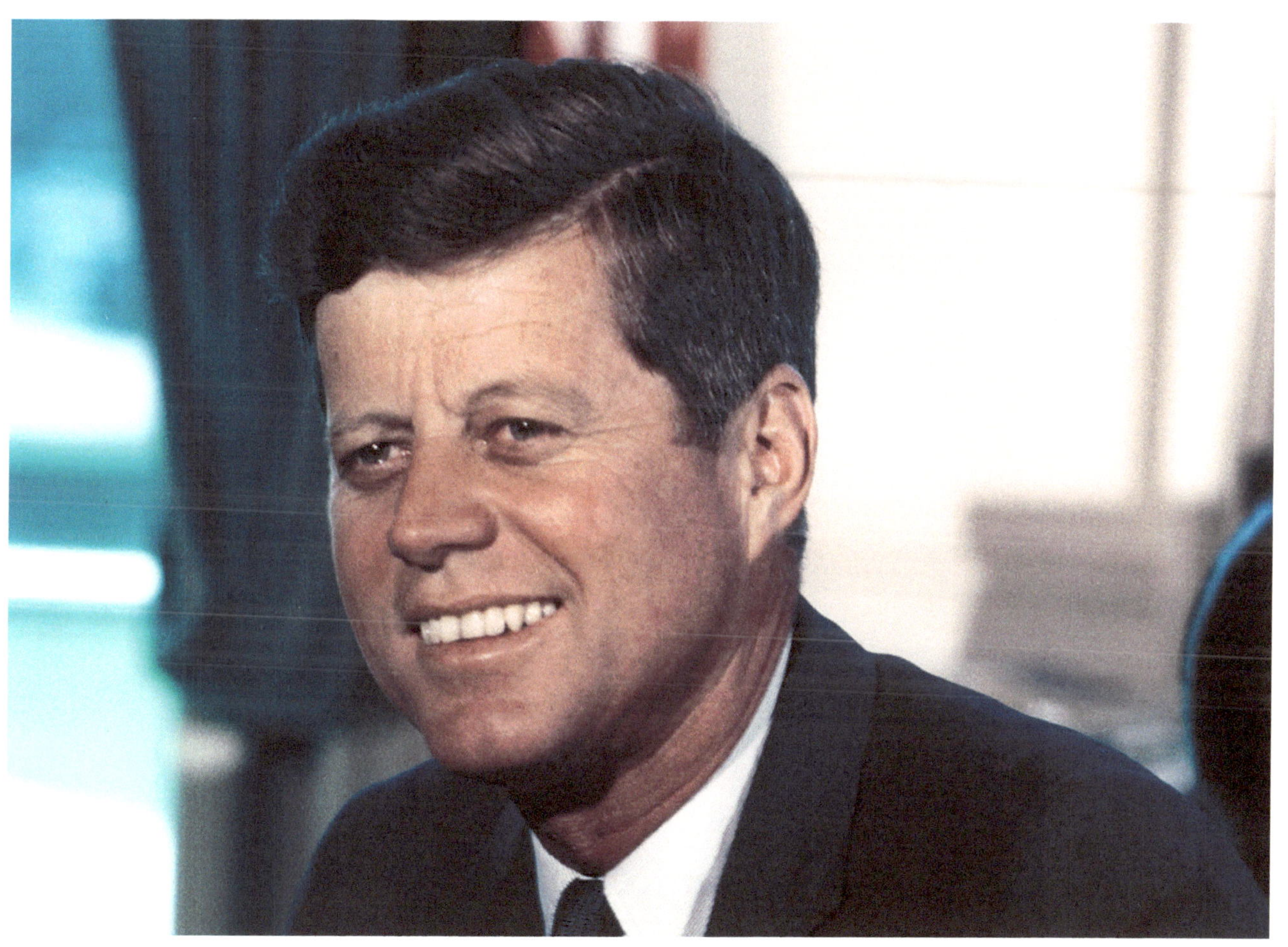

John F. Kennedy

Famous Icons

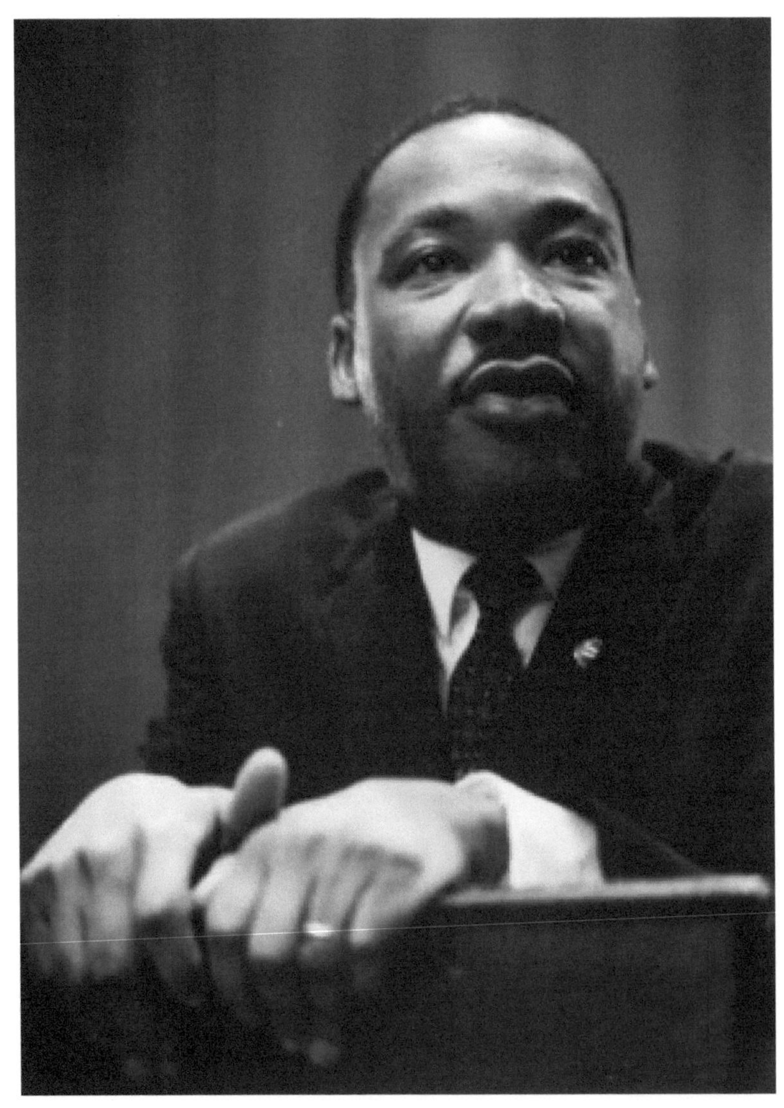

Martin Luther King Jr.

Airliners

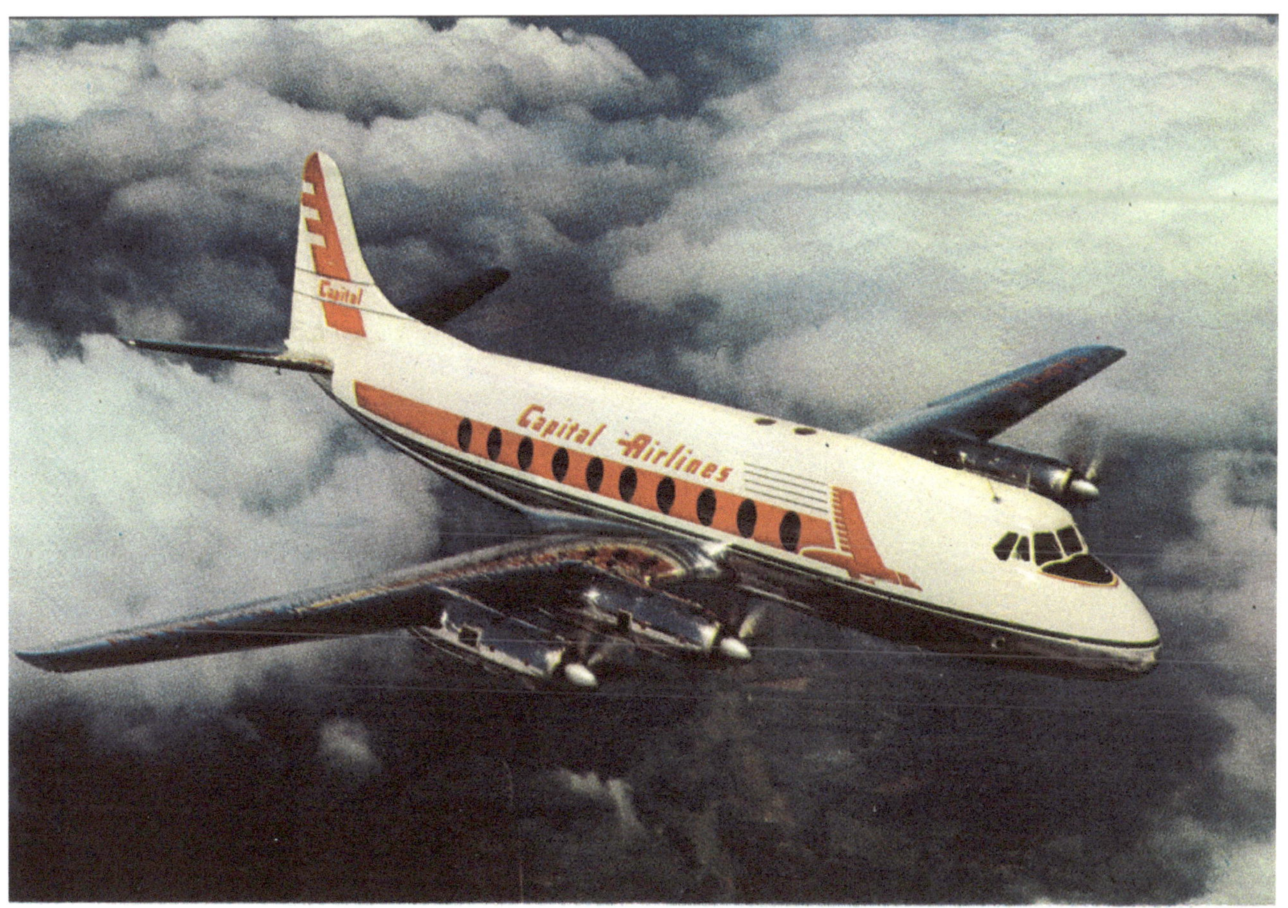

THE *CAPITAL VISCOUNT* .... *A NEW CONCEPT IN FLIGHT*

Capital Airlines

Airliners

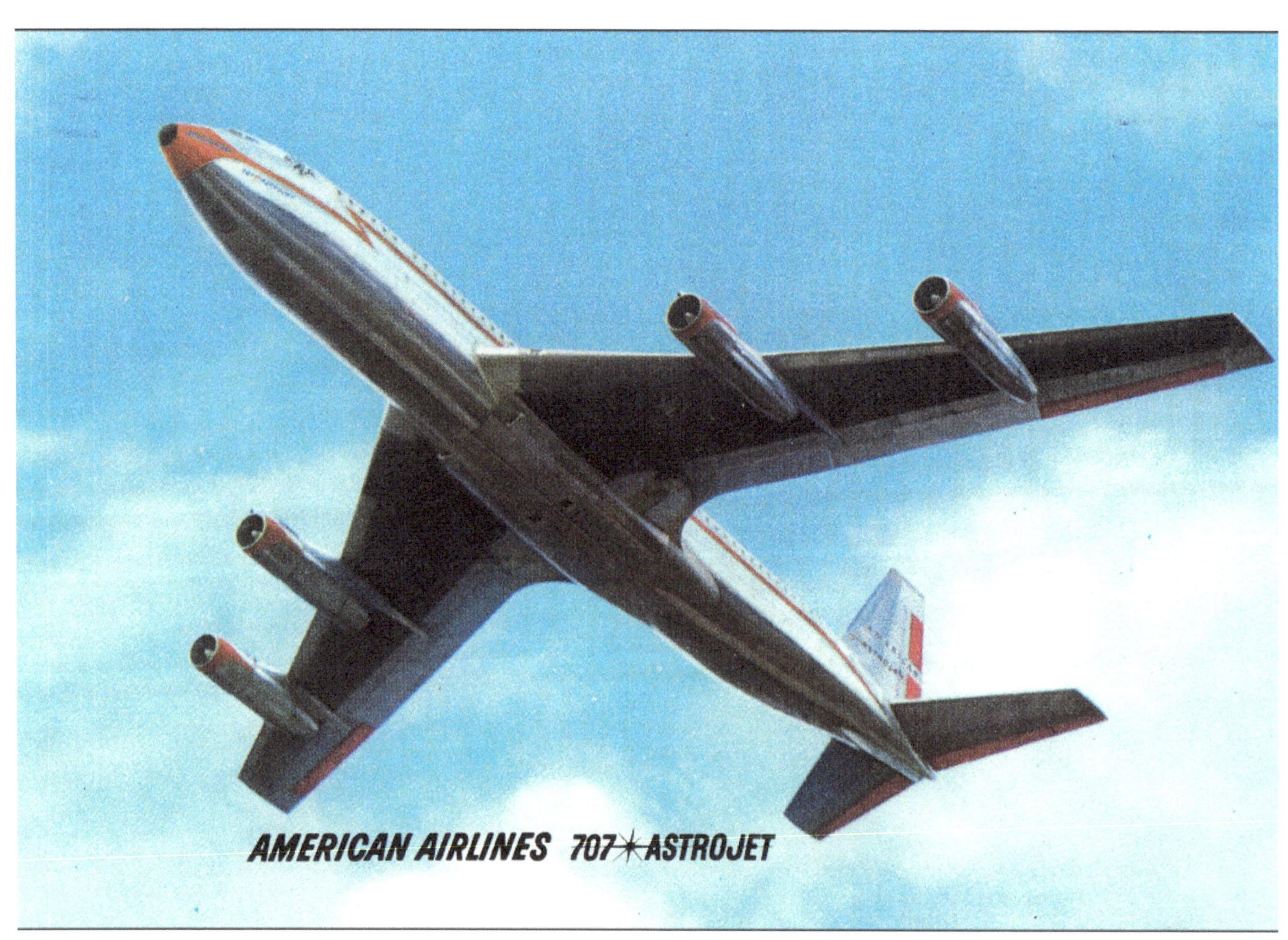

American Airlines 707

Airliners

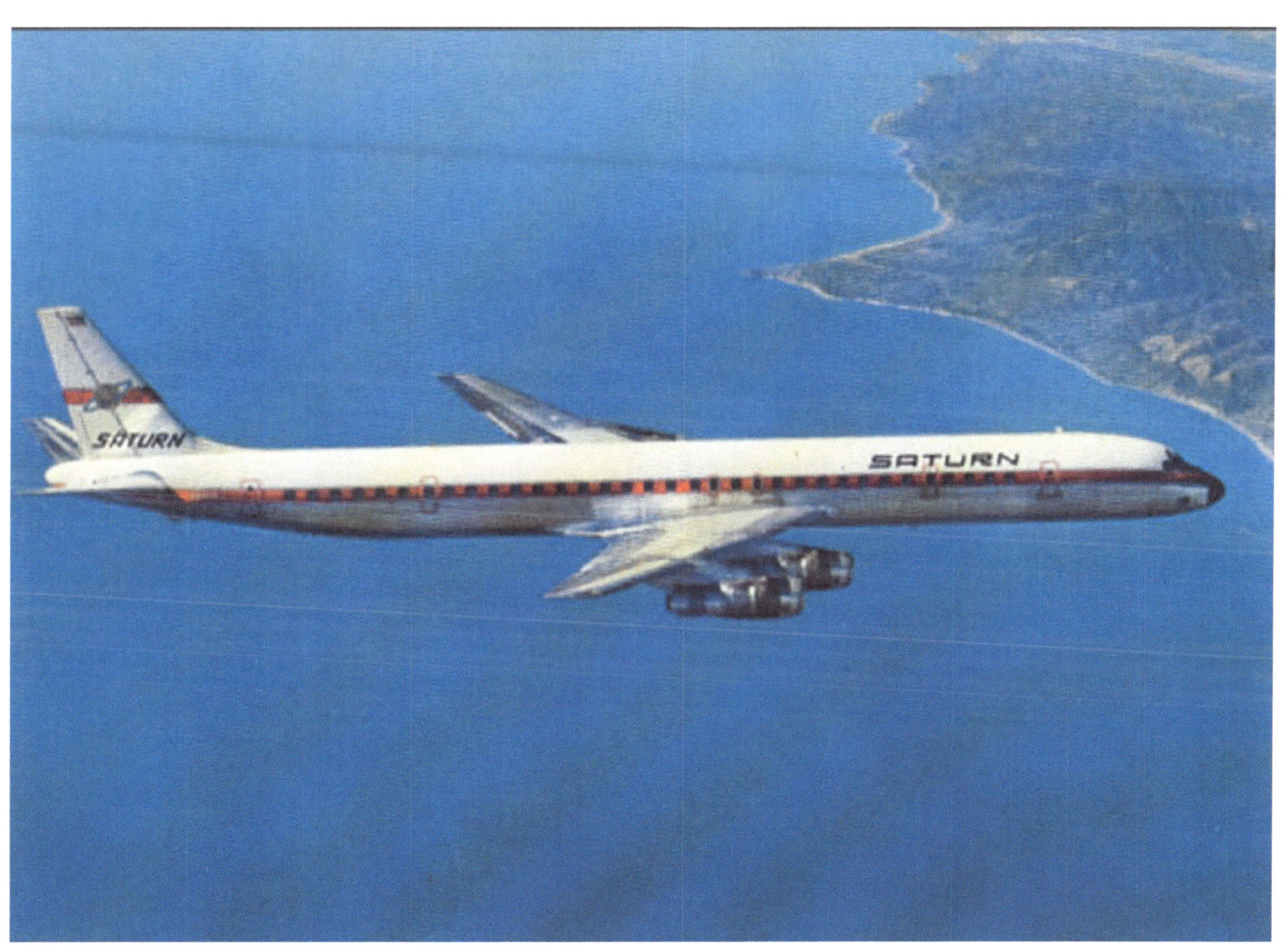

Saturn Airlines

Vietnam War Photos

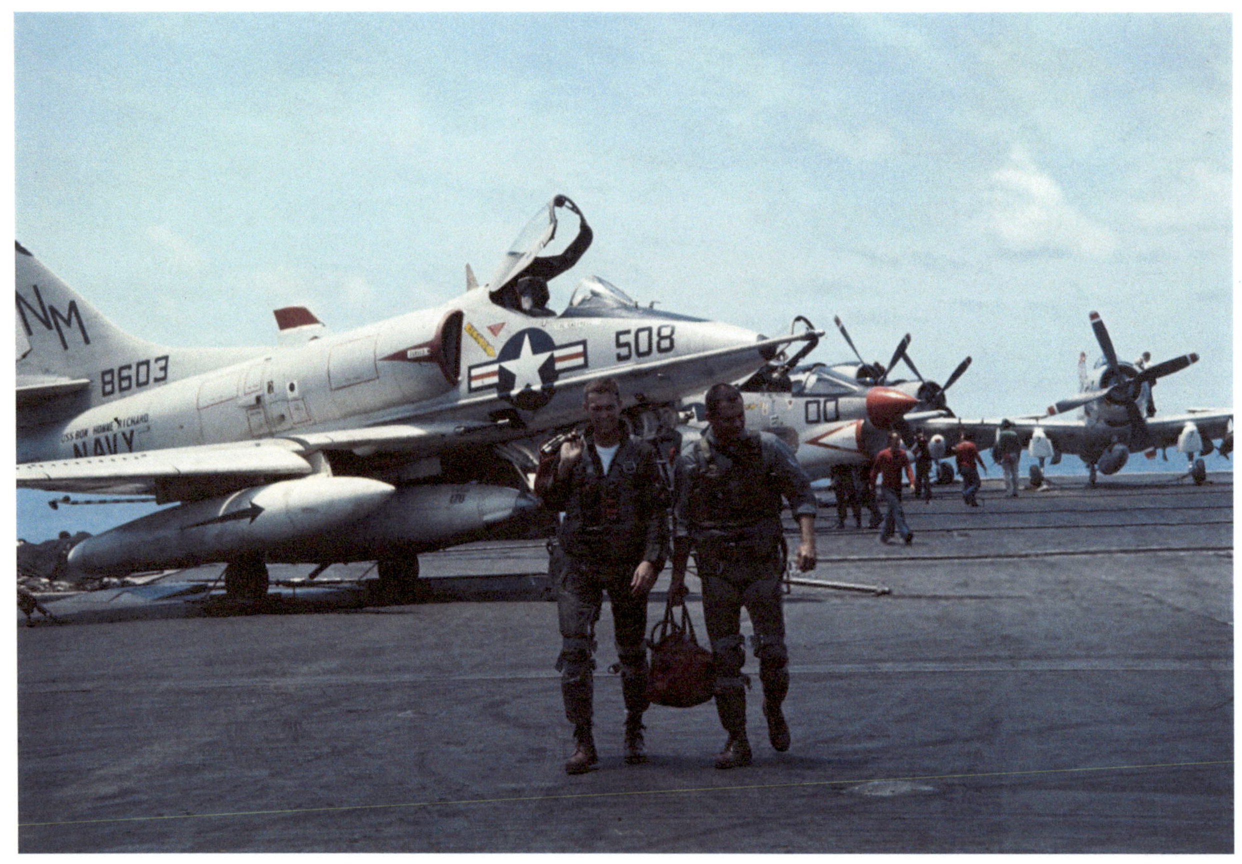

Navy Soldiers Walking with Bombers in Background

Vietnam War Photos

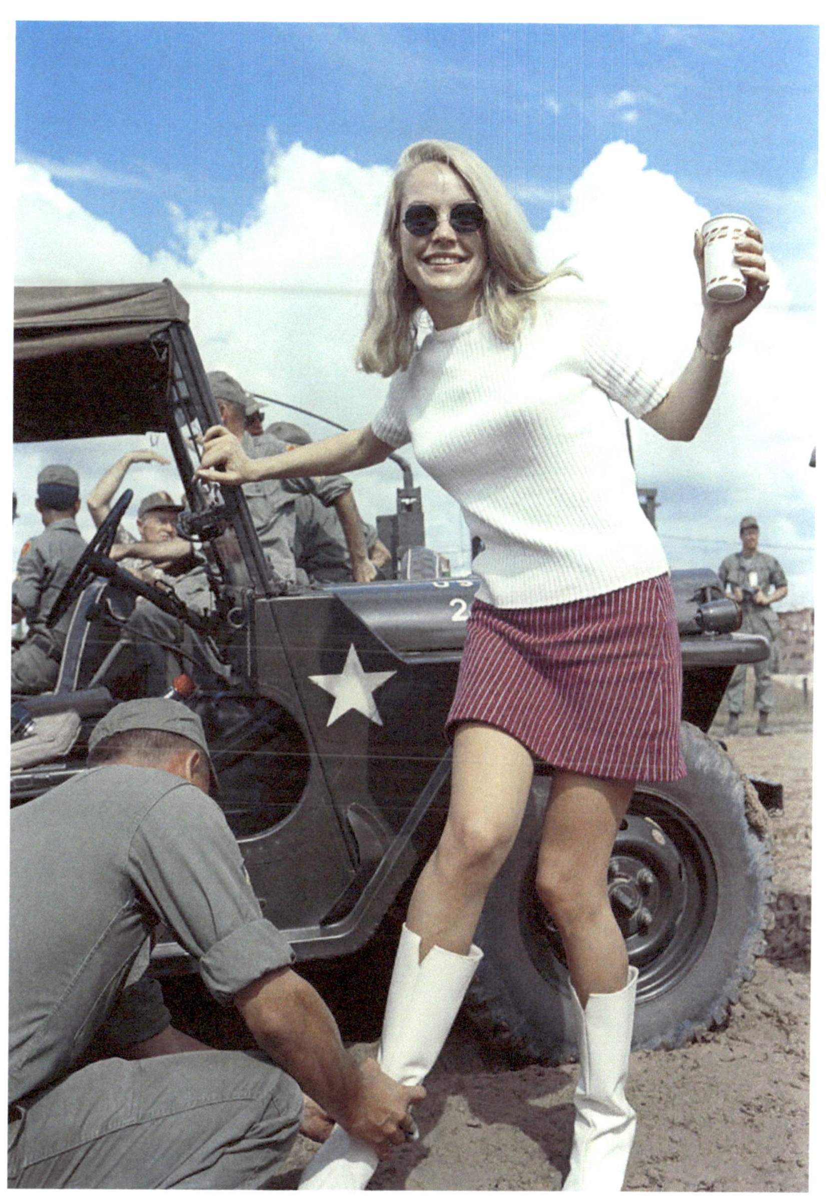

Chris Noel in South Vietnam entertaining soldiers

Vietnam War Photos

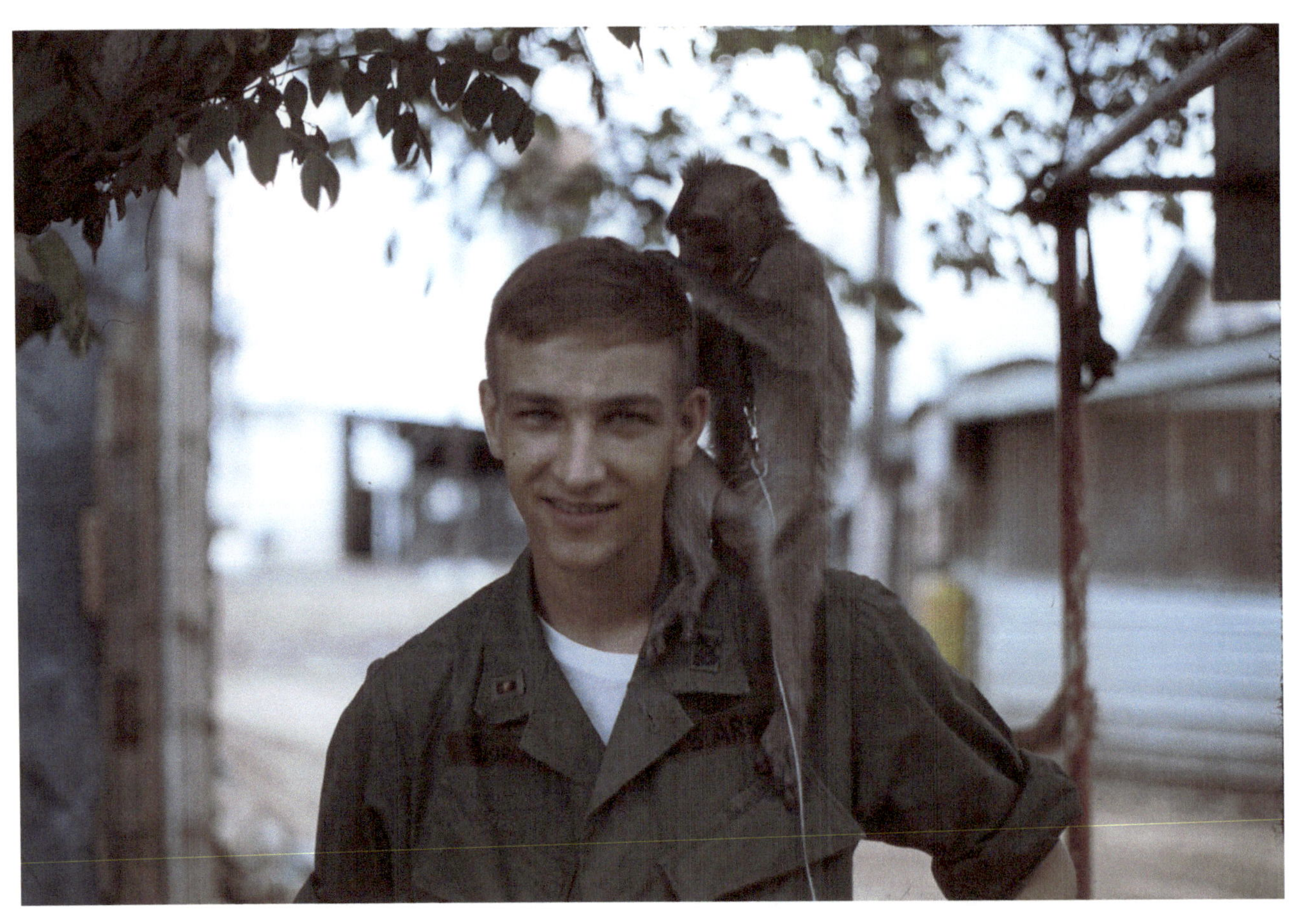

Outlaws & Mavericks /175th AHC - U.S. Army

Kitchen Styles

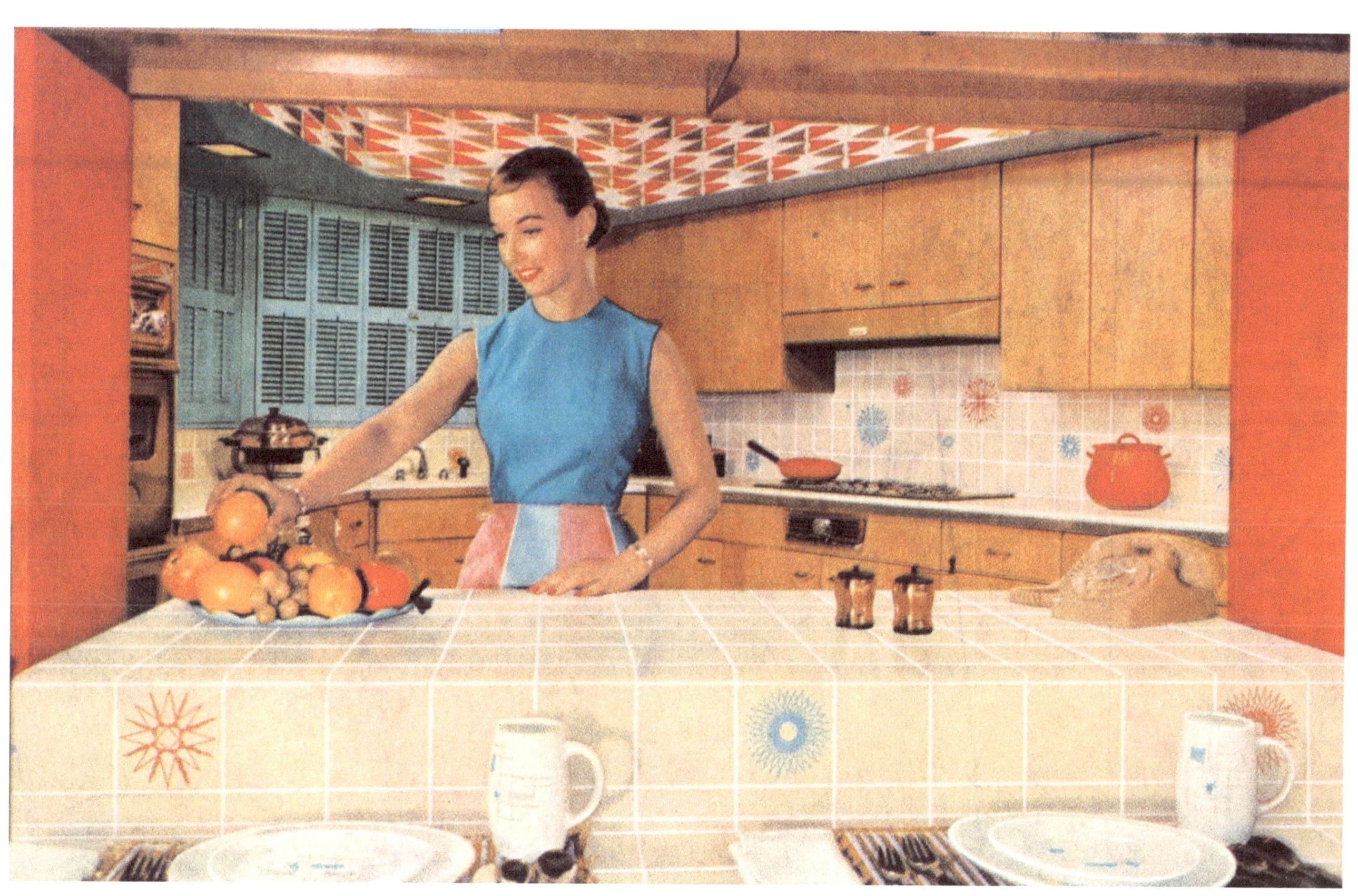

Kitchen Styles

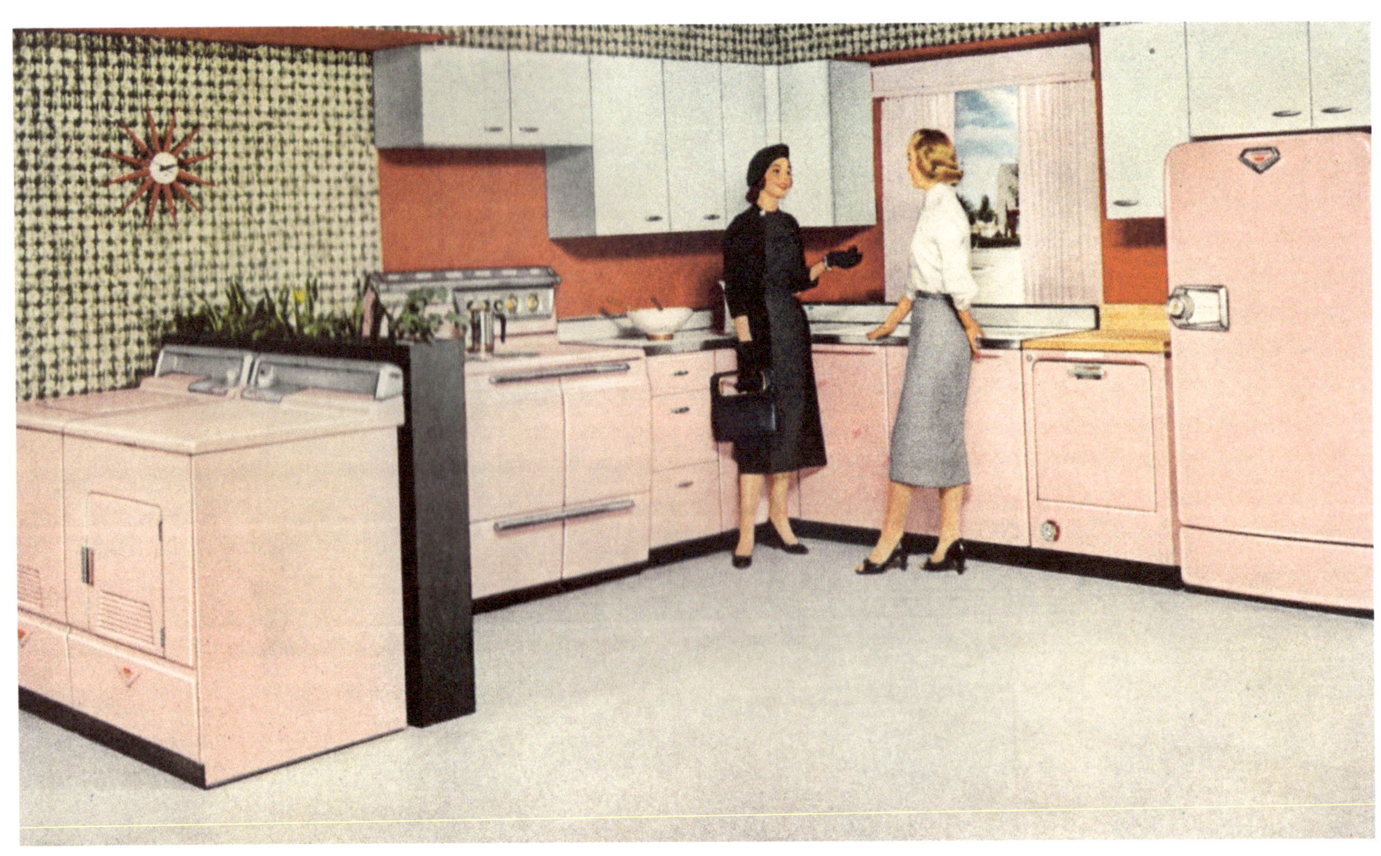

Kitchen Styles

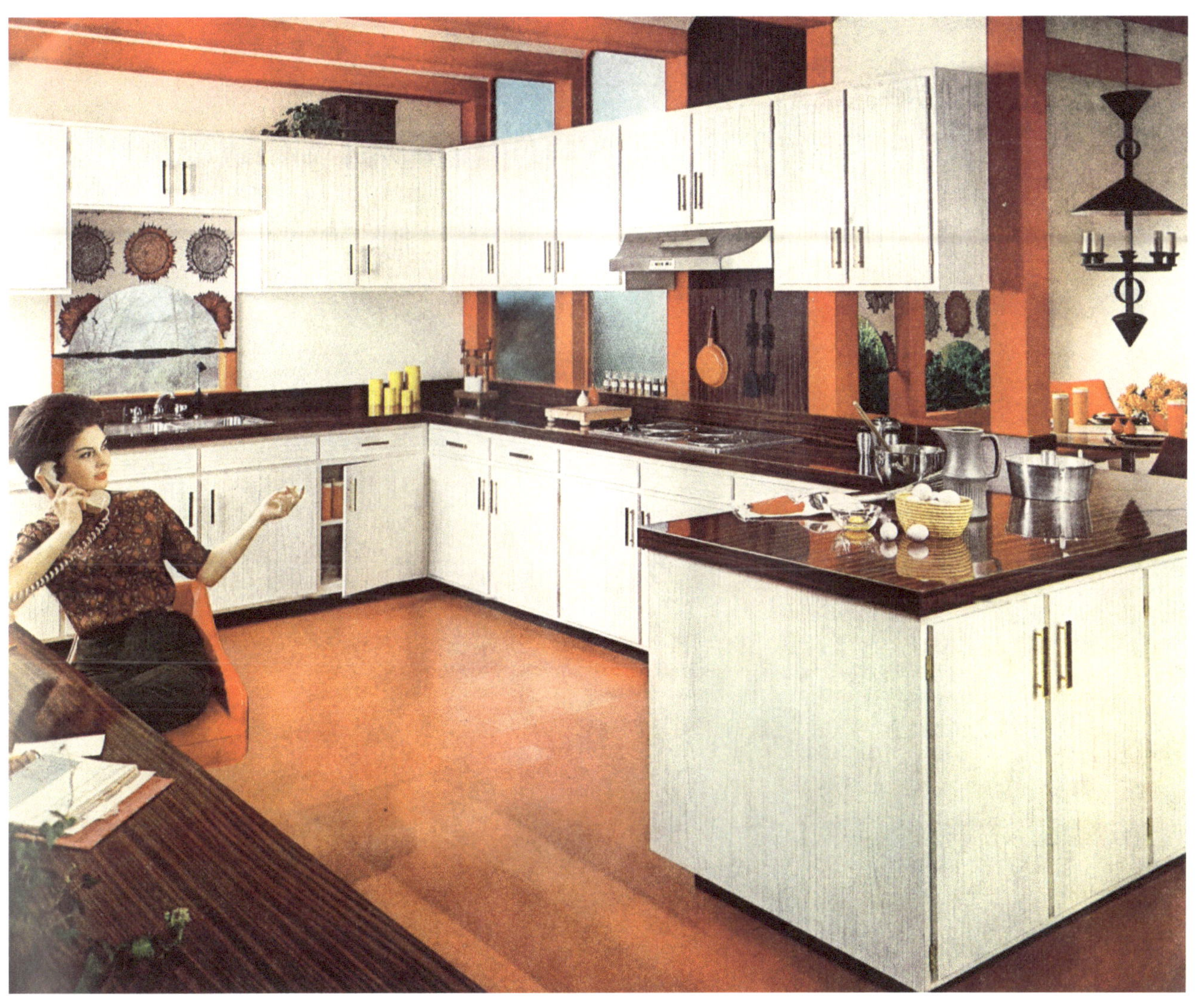

Women's Fashion

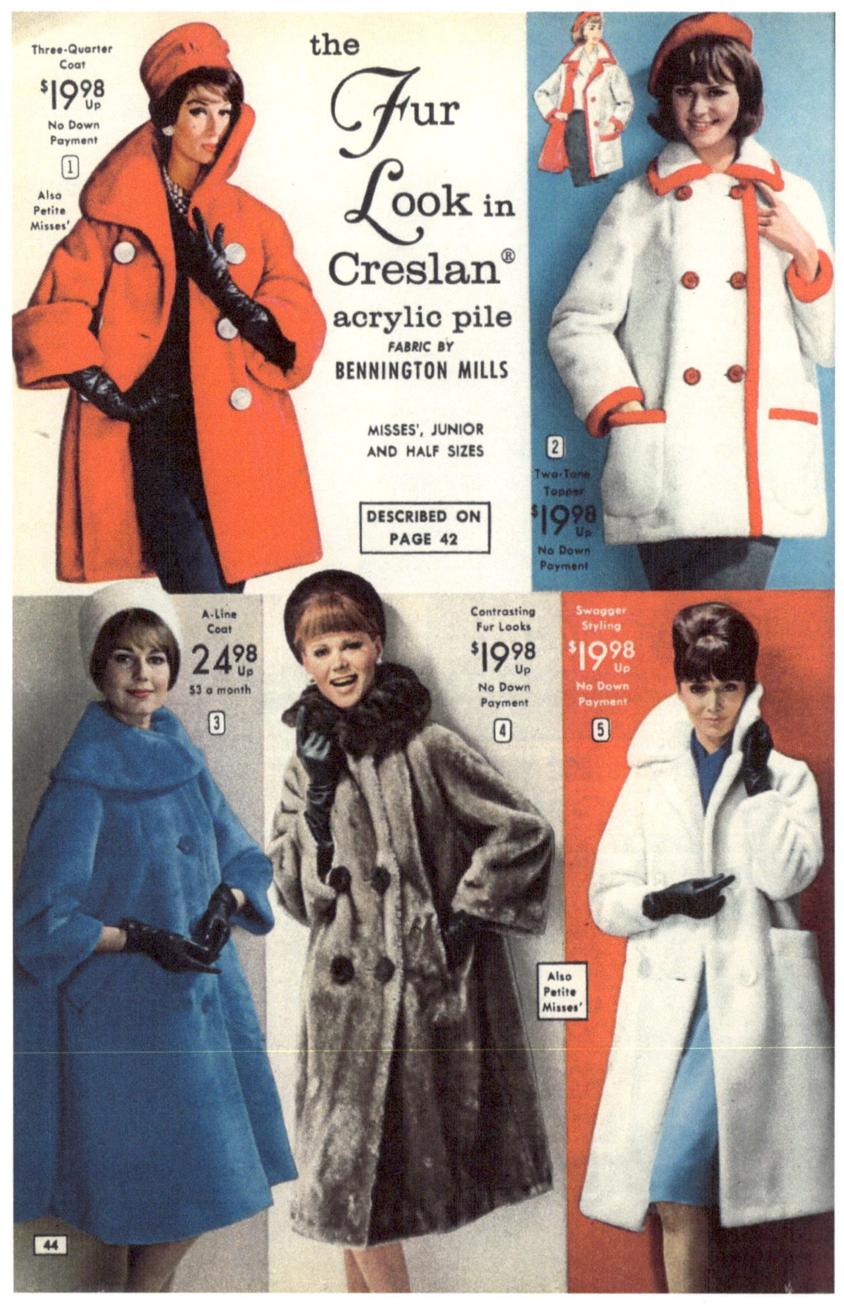

Women's Fashion

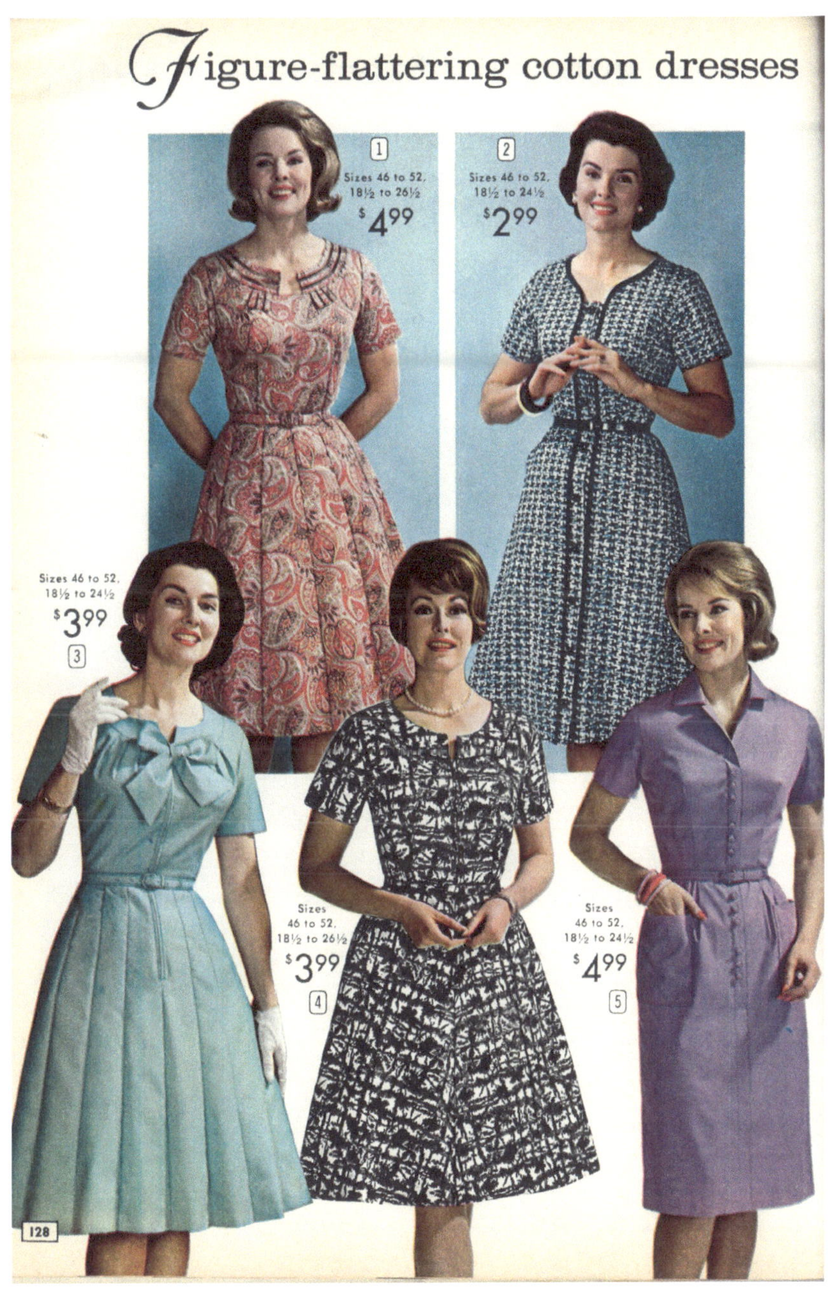

Women's Fashion

Tweed with Suedecloth
$8 98 Up 2 Pc.
6
Also Juniors'
Fur-Trimmed Laminate
$14 98 Up 2 Pc.
7
SUITS
for thrifty you
MISSES' AND HALF SIZES
DESCRIBED ON PAGE 42
Fur-Crowned Walking Suit
$19 98 Up 2 Pc.
No Down Payment
10
Laminated Crepe
$13 98 Up 2 Pc.
8
Also Juniors
Looped-Weave Wool -Nylon
$10 98 Up 2 Pc.
9
Also Juniors
45

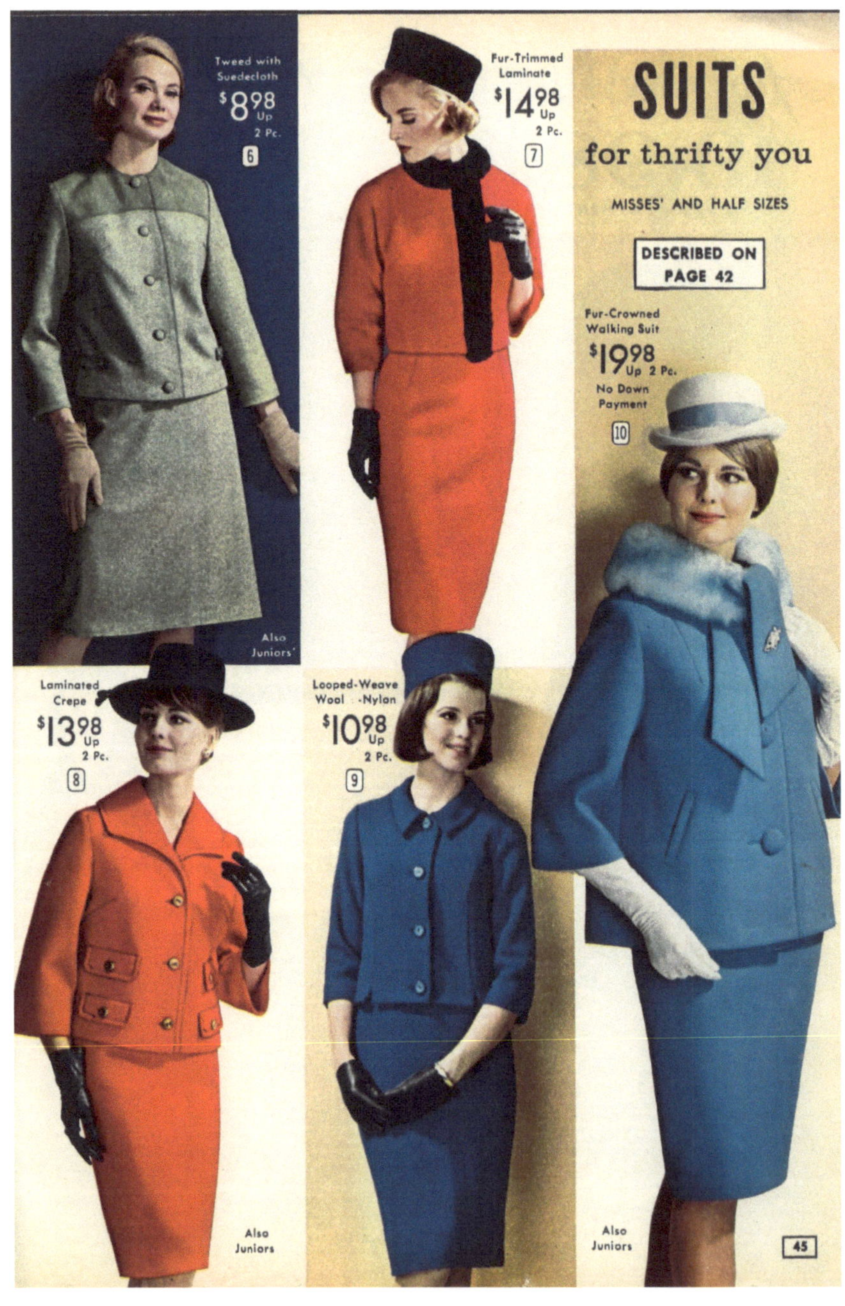

Living Room Décor

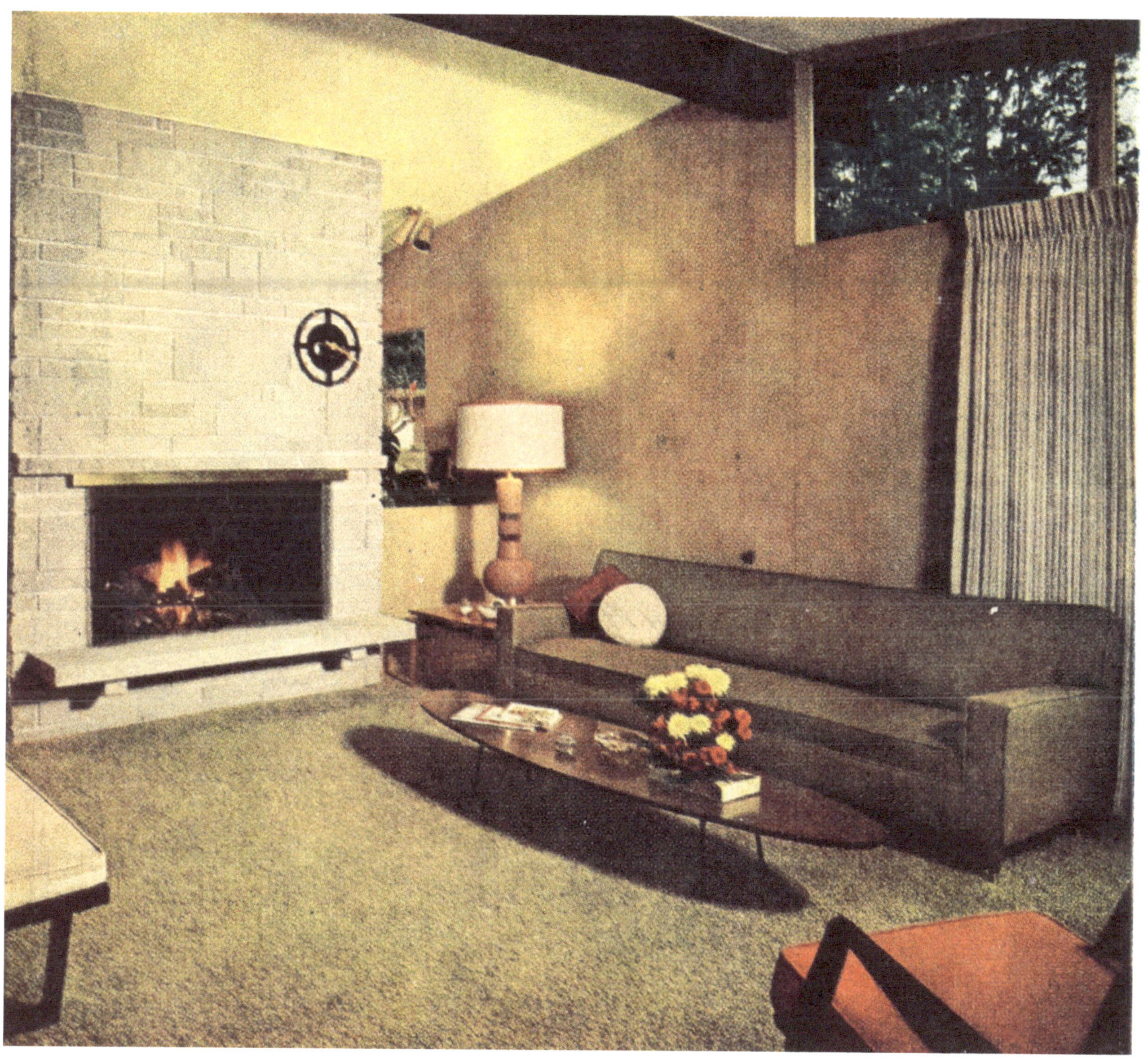

Living Room Décor

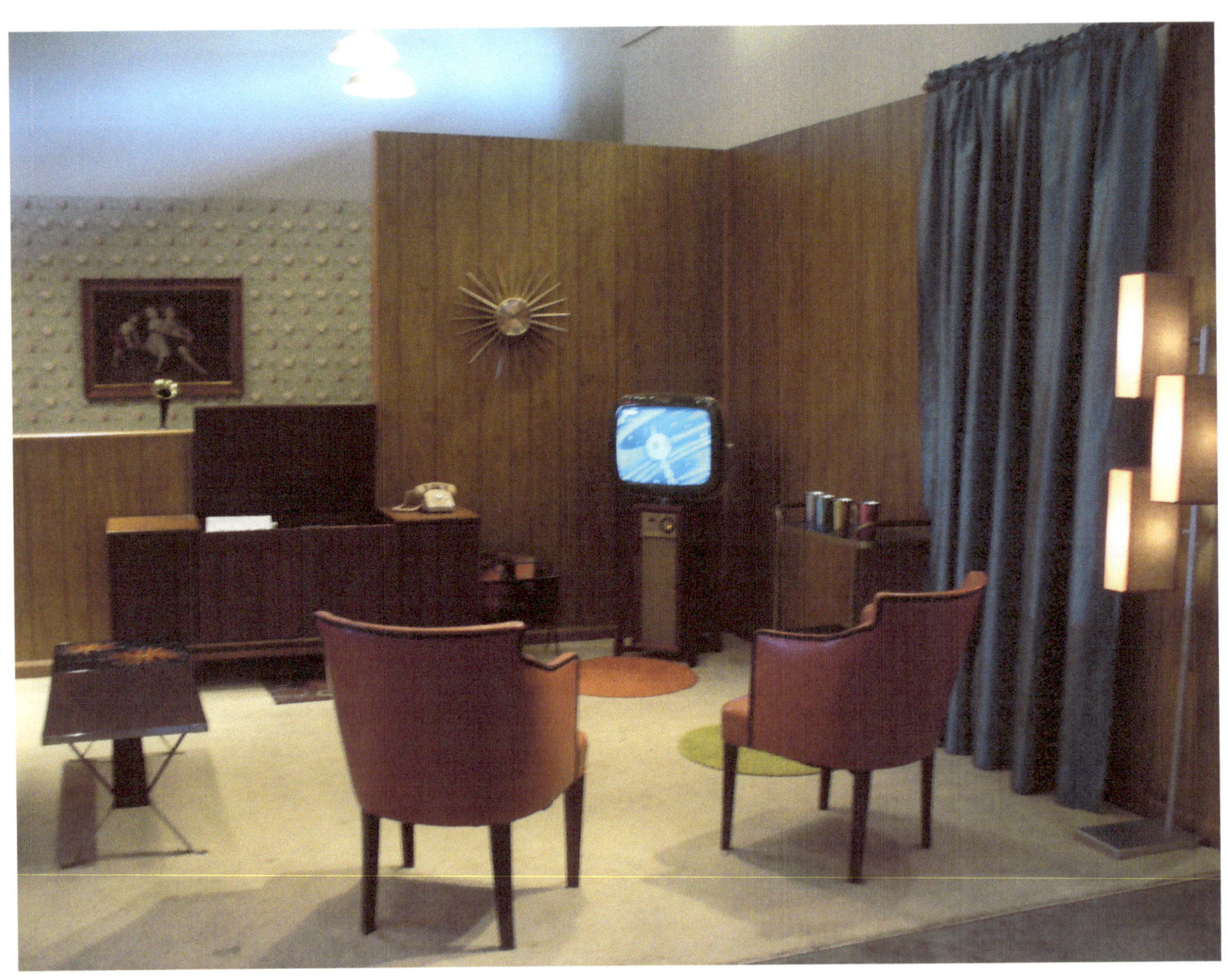

Living Room Décor

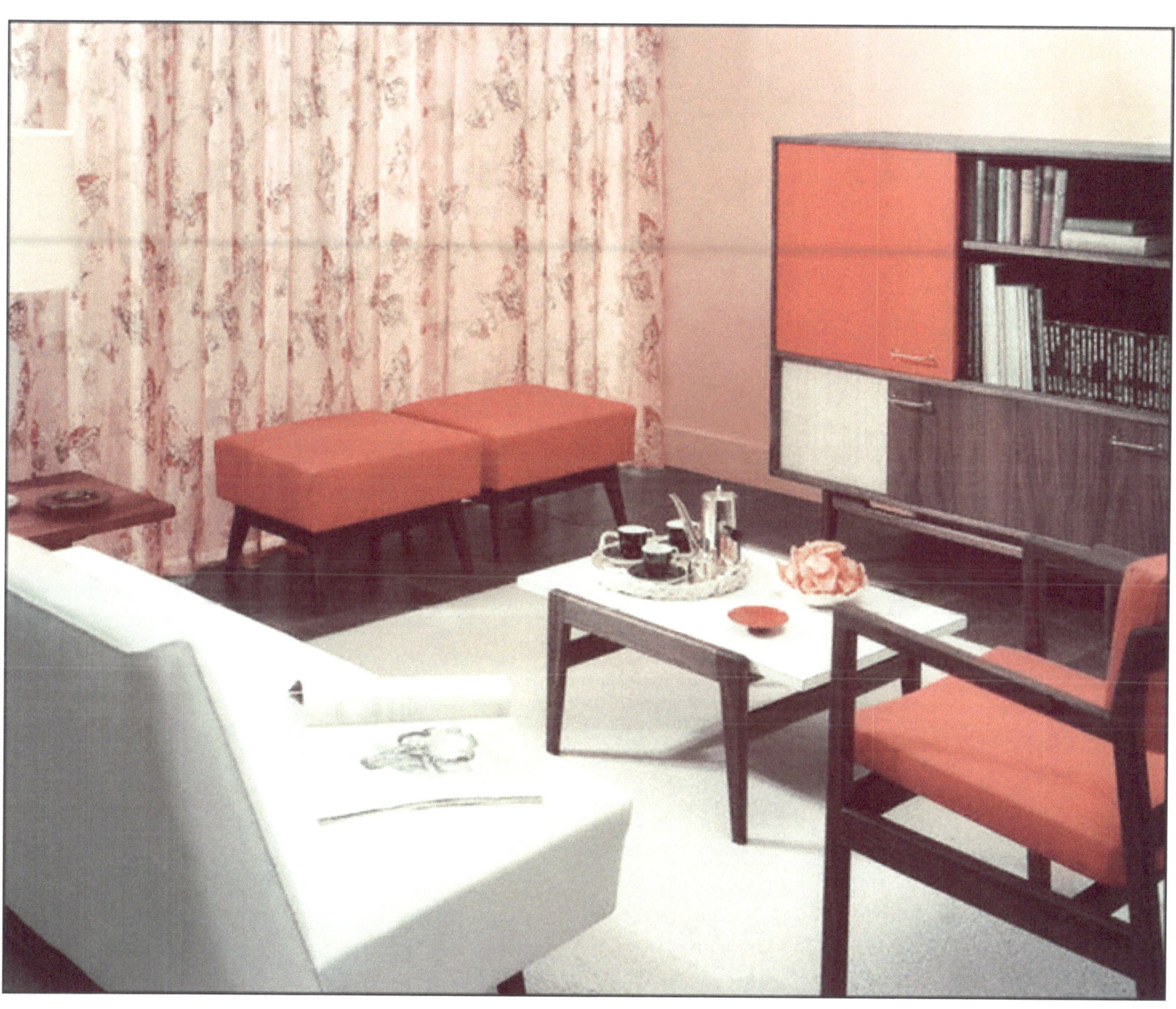

Families

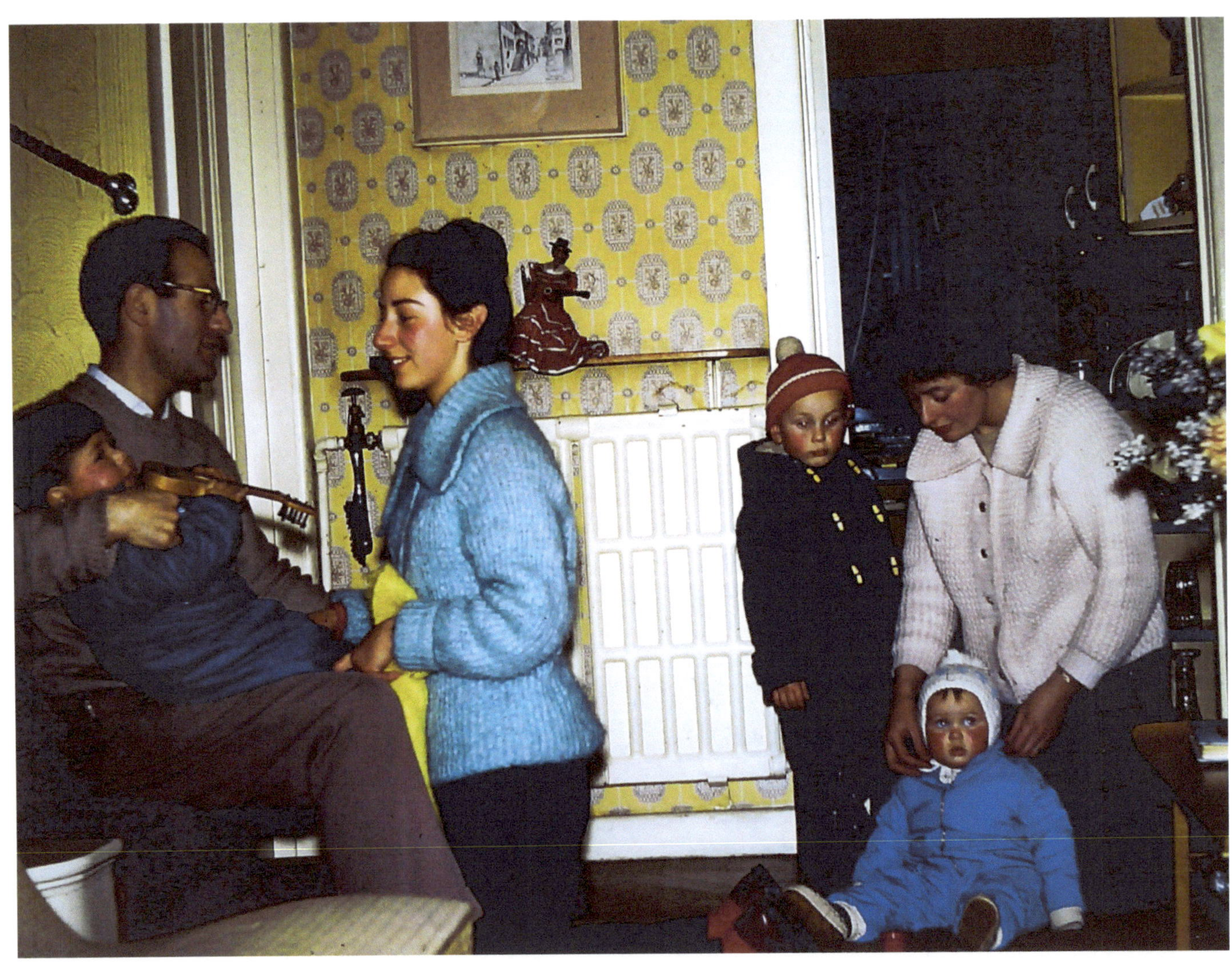

Families

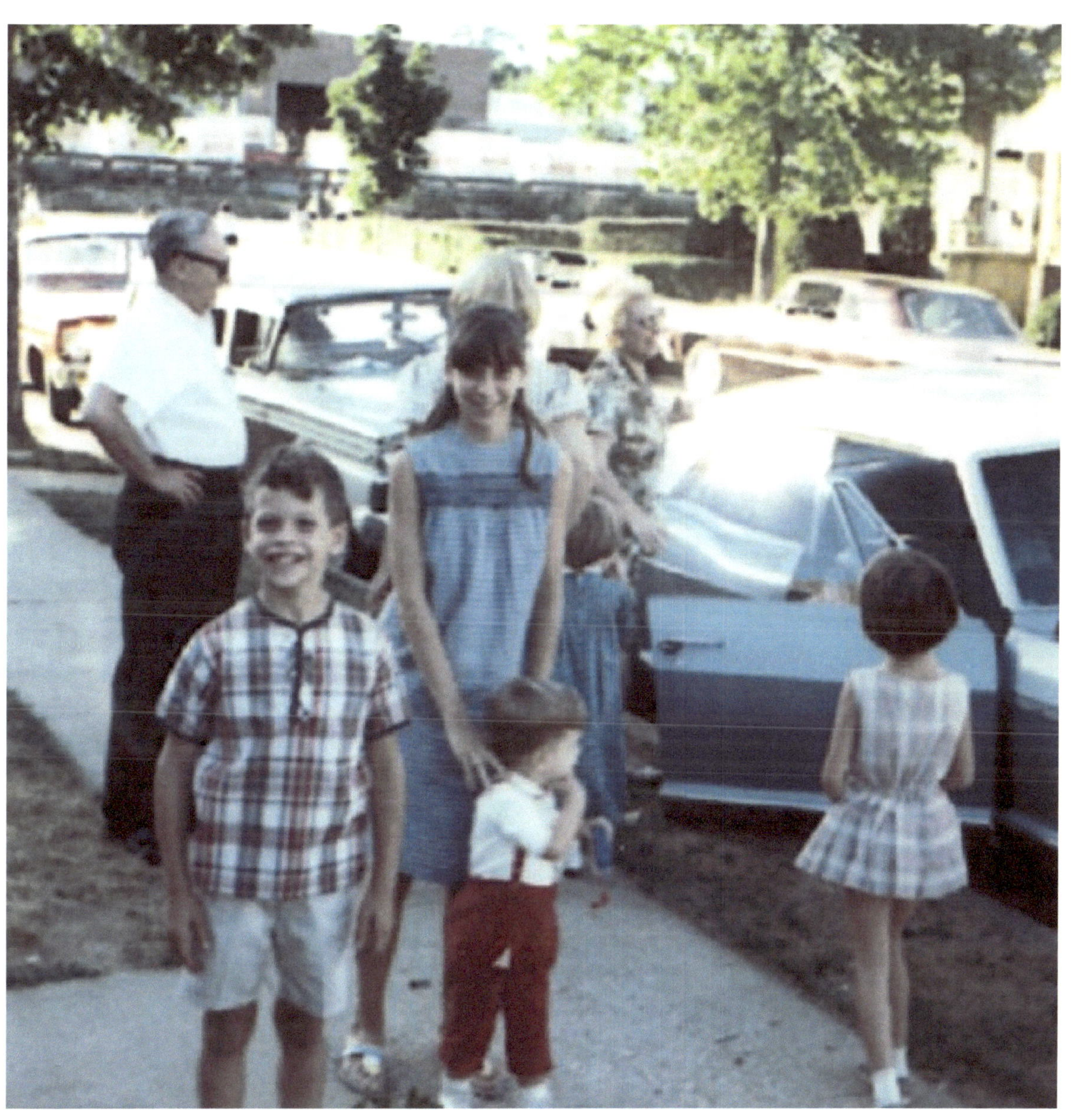

Families

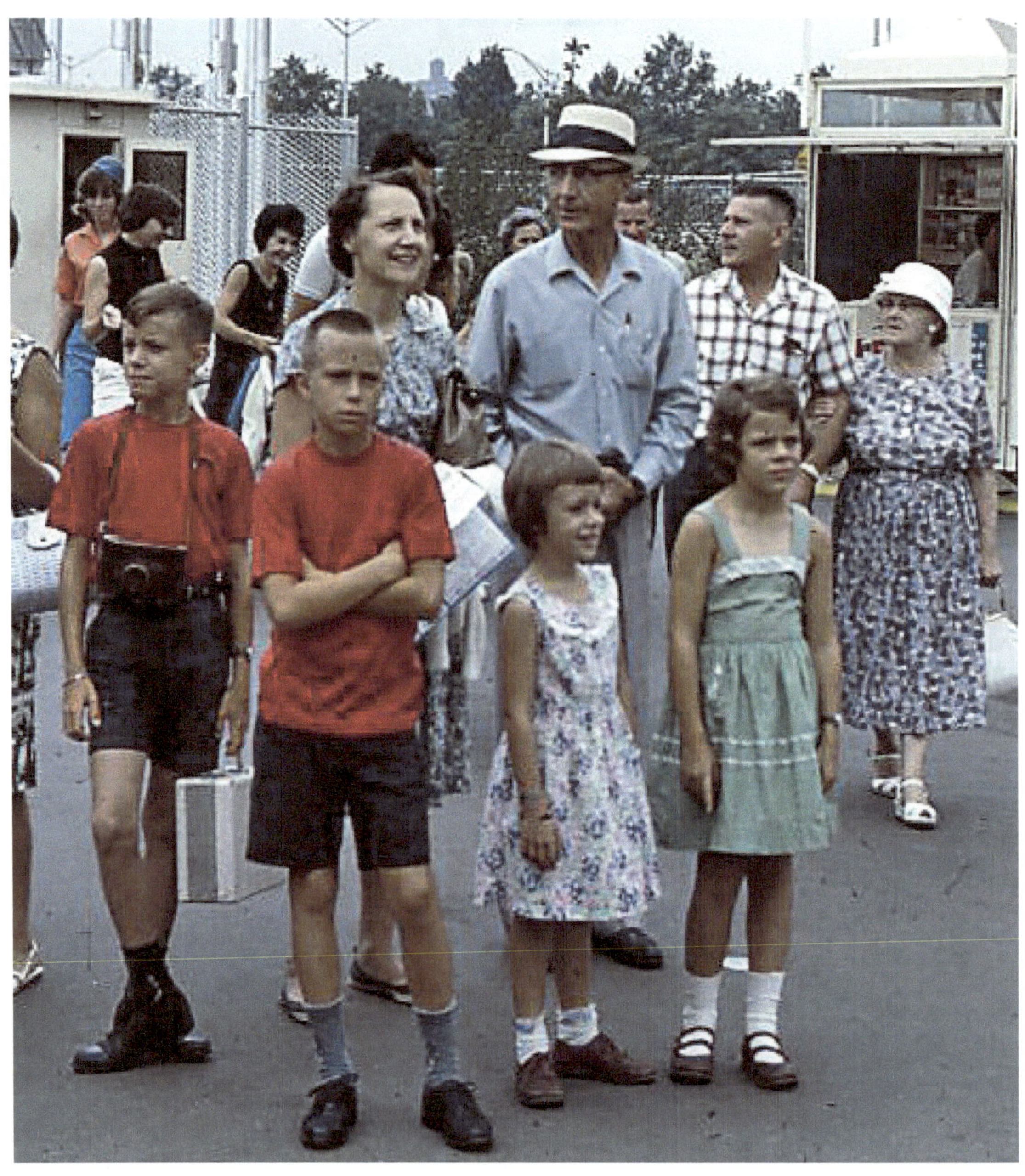

Famous Places

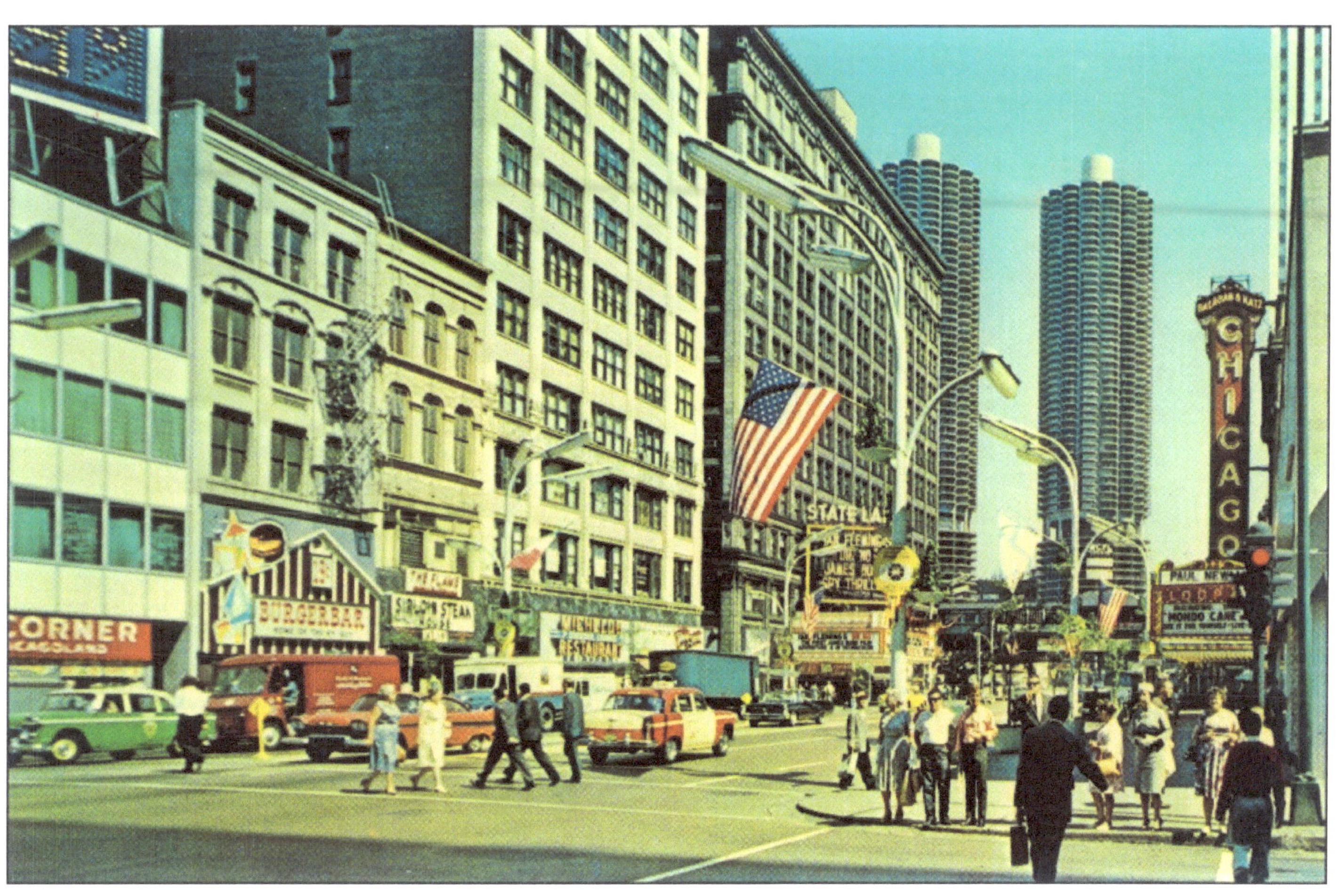

State Street Randolph, Chicago 64

Famous Places

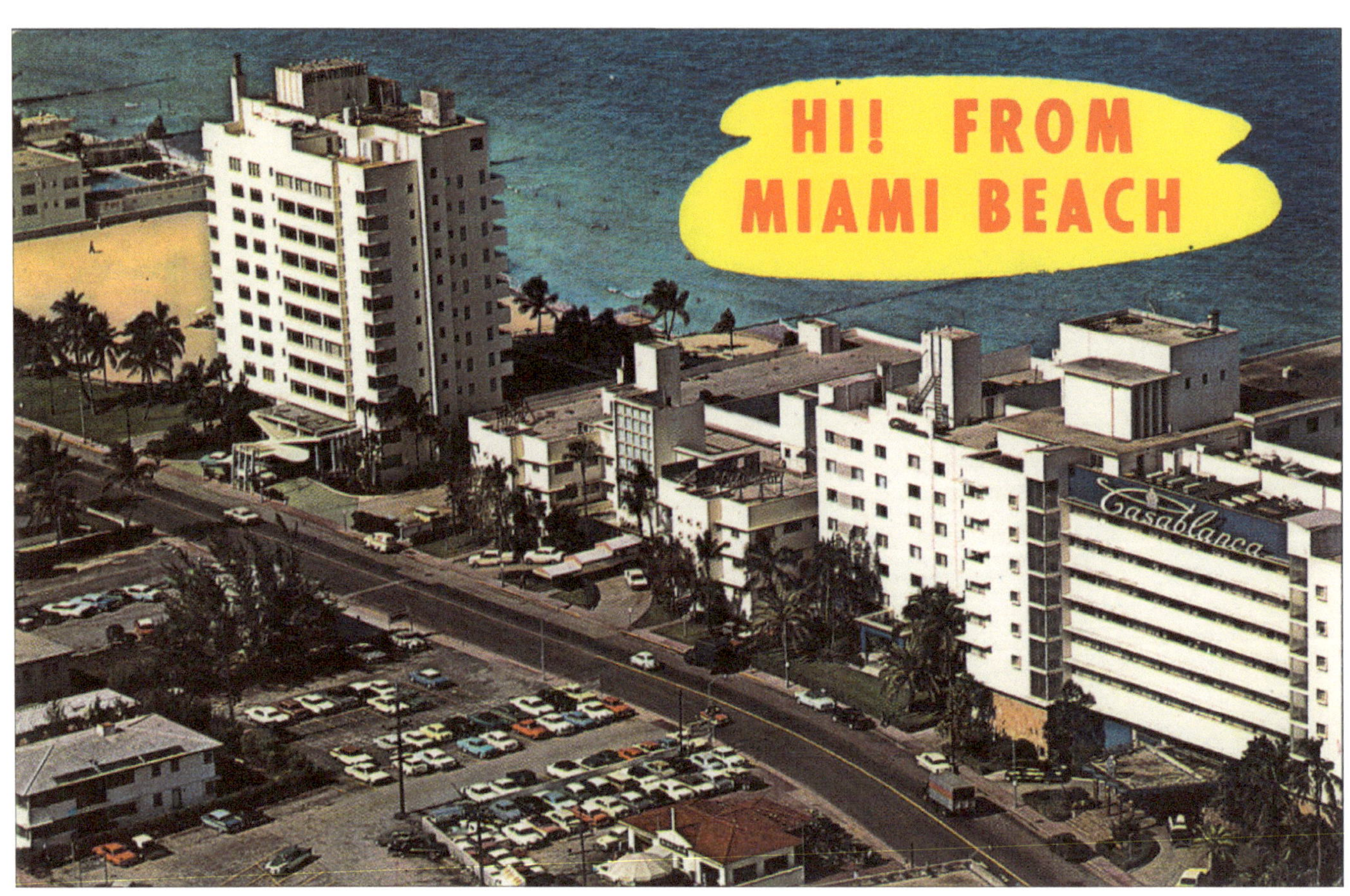

miami beach florida 1964

Famous Places

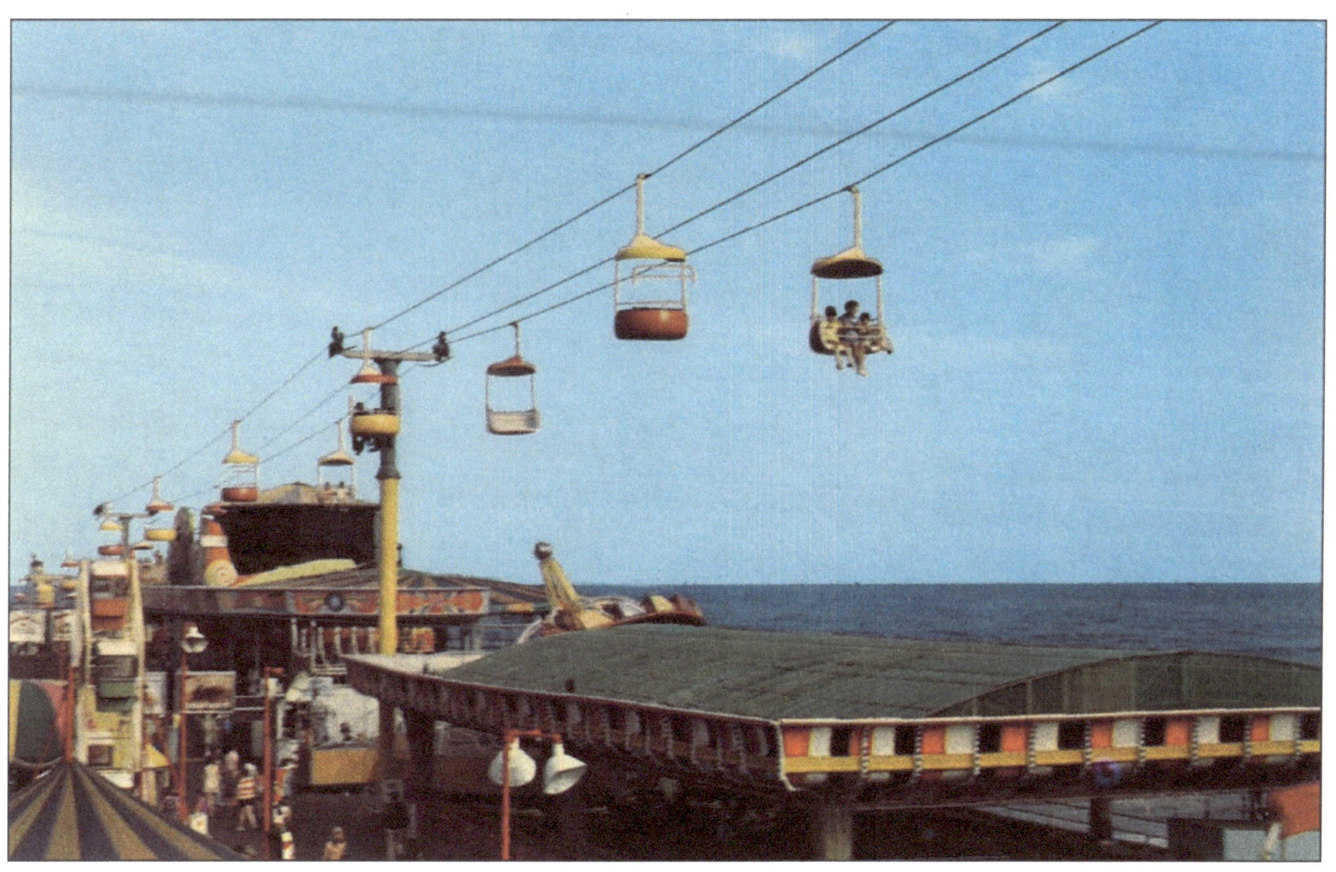

Midway on Casino Pier & Rides - Seaside Park
New Jersey

Famous Places

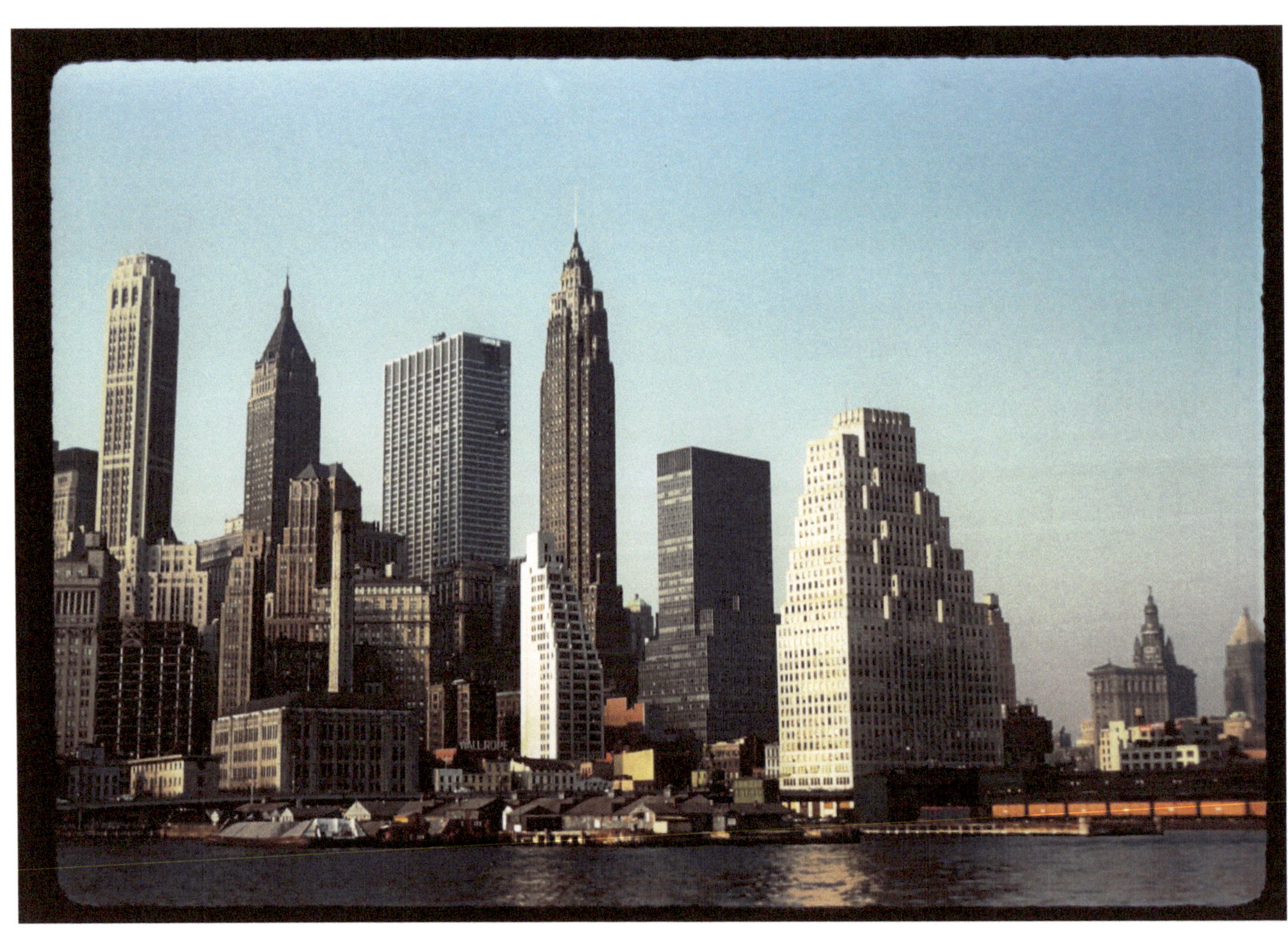

Newyork in 1960s

Easter In The 60s

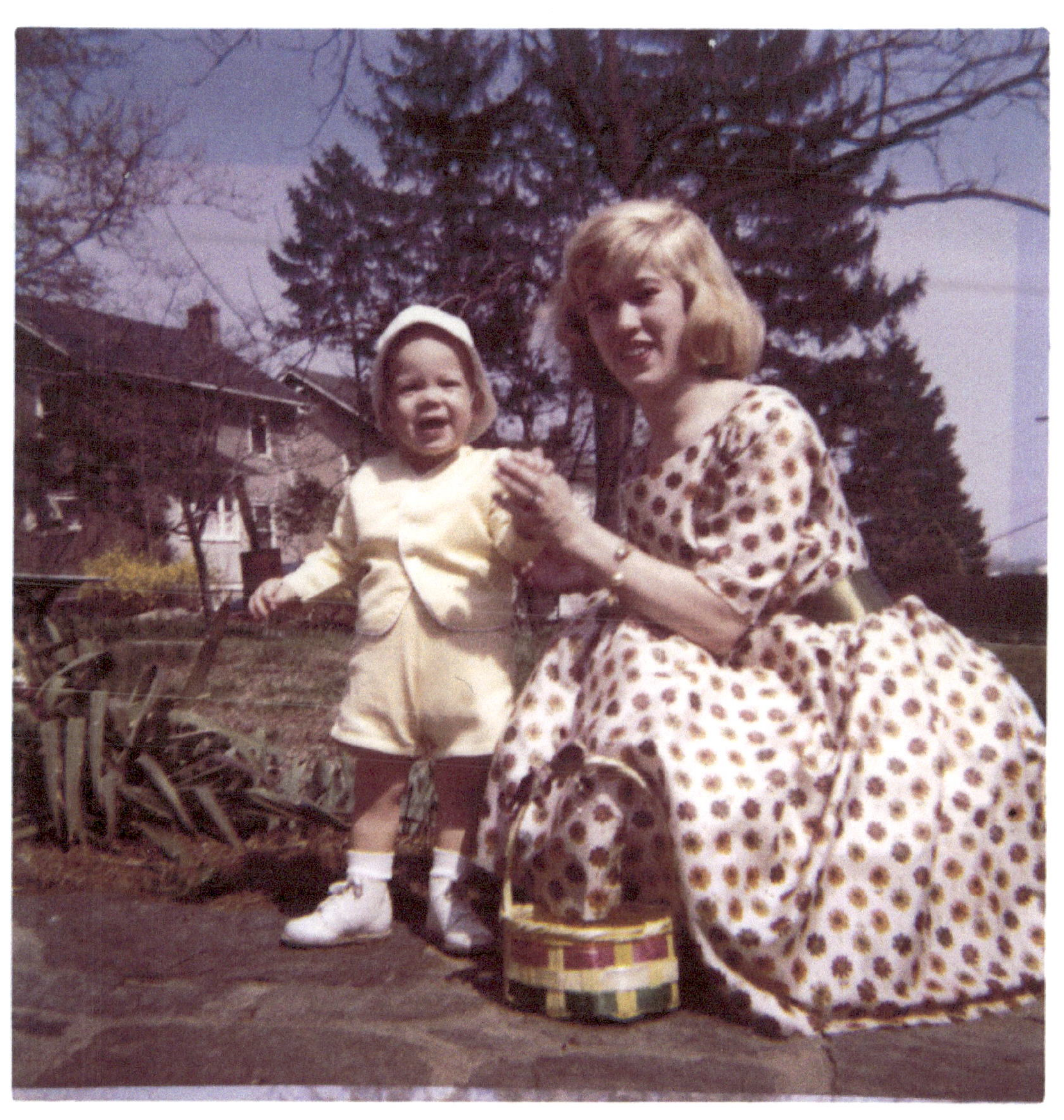

Christmas in The 60s

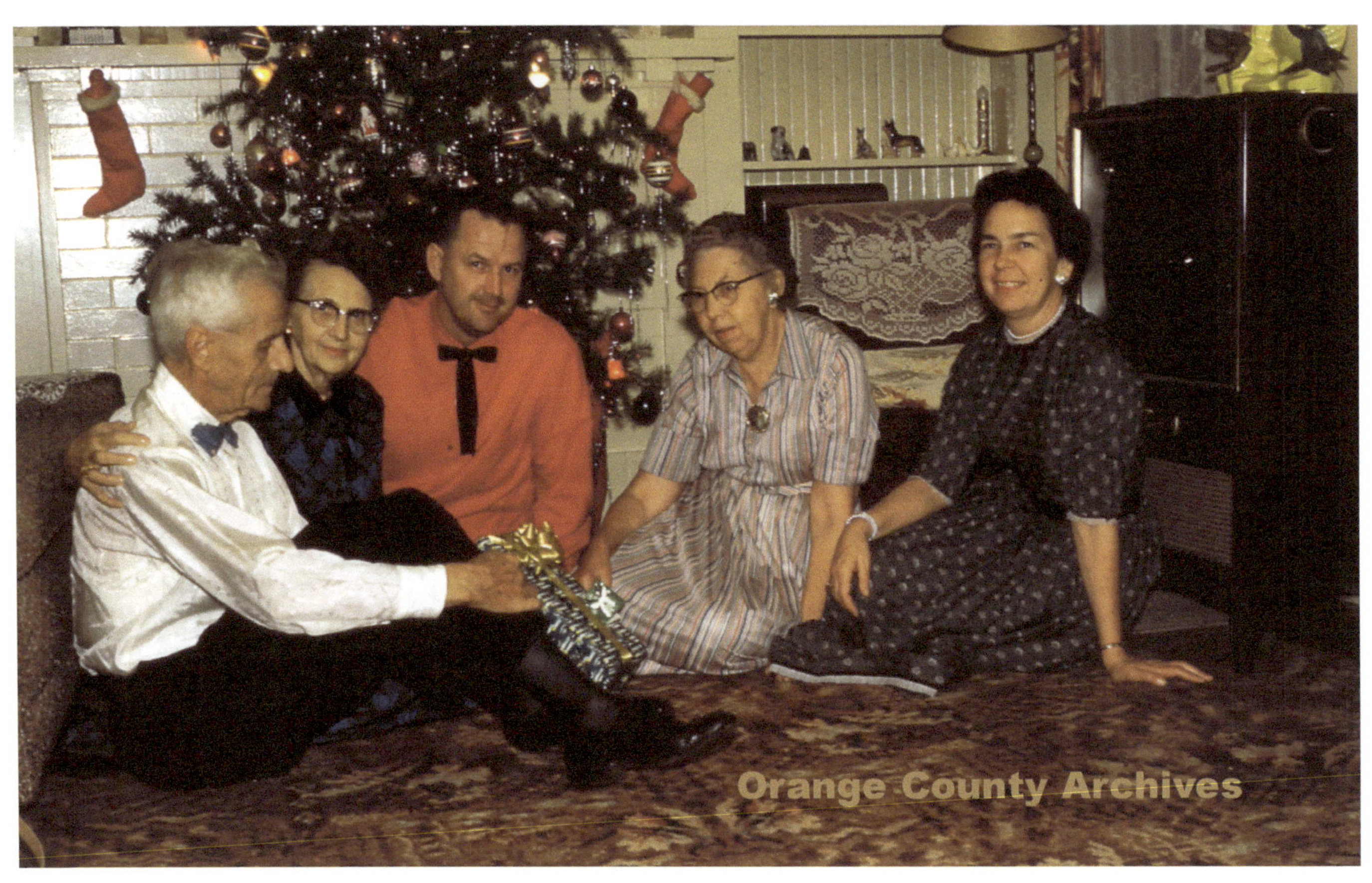

Christmas in The 60s

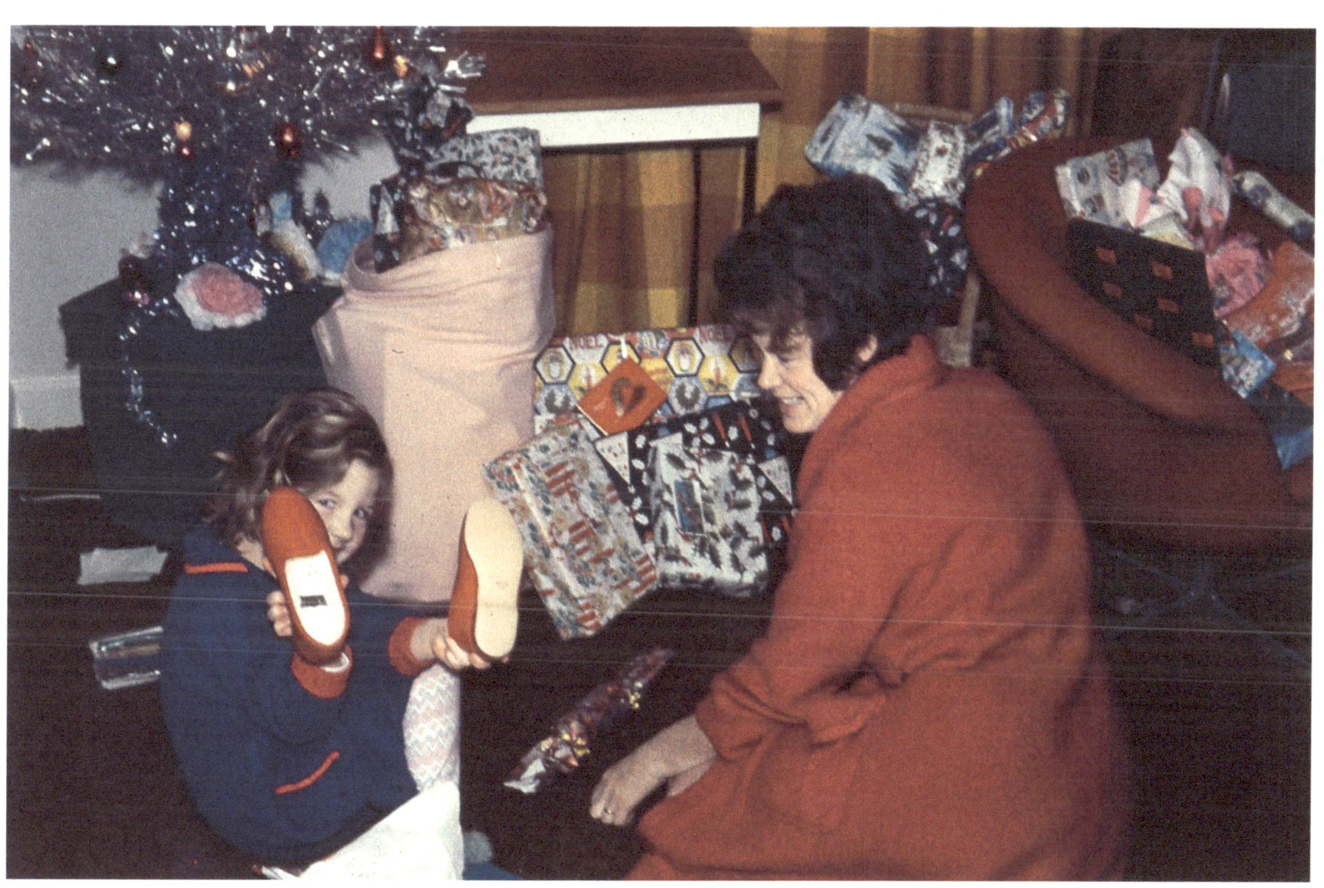

Acknowledgement

Page No. I Author/s I Title I Source I License

Children's Advertisement I 1950sUnlimited
Kraft Marshmallow Creme 1960 I https://www.flickr.com/photos/blakta2/8194840337/
Attribution 2.0 Generic (CC BY 2.0)

Children's Advertisement I 1950sUnlimited
Bell Telephone System I https://www.flickr.com/photos/blakta2/8176816197/
Attribution 2.0 Generic (CC BY 2.0)

Refreshing Drinks I 1950sUnlimited
1960 7UP I https://www.flickr.com/photos/blakta2/8180214230/
Attribution 2.0 Generic (CC BY 2.0)

Refreshing Drinks I 1950sUnlimited
Sprite 1967 I https://www.flickr.com/photos/blakta2/8238519503/
Attribution 2.0 Generic (CC BY 2.0)

Advertisements for Women I 1950sUnlimited
1965MaxFactor I https://www.flickr.com/photos/blakta2/8174046275/
Attribution 2.0 Generic (CC BY 2.0)

Advertisements for Women I 1950sUnlimited
Professional Prell I https://www.flickr.com/photos/blakta2/8201573467/
Attribution 2.0 Generic (CC BY 2.0)

Best Cars Of The 60s I Andrew Bone (andreboeni)
BMC Mini (early 1960s) I https://www.flickr.com/photos/andreboeni/26089130368/
Attribution 2.0 Generic (CC BY 2.0)

Best Cars Of The 60s I 1950sUnlimited
1966 Ford Fairlane I https://www.flickr.com/photos/blakta2/8219463367/
Attribution 2.0 Generic (CC BY 2.0)

Best Cars Of The 60s I 1950sUnlimited
1960 Dodge Polara and Matador I https://www.flickr.com/photos/blakta2/8286032185/
Attribution 2.0 Generic (CC BY 2.0)

Top Actors I Insomnia Cured Here (tom-margie)
Stagecoach (1939) I https://www.flickr.com/photos/tom-margie/2075500063/
Attribution-ShareAlike 2.0 Generic (CC BY-SA 2.0)

Top Actors I Insomnia Cured Here (tom-margie)
Paul Newman 1925-2008 I https://www.flickr.com/photos/tom-margie/1548698548/
Attribution-ShareAlike 2.0 Generic (CC BY-SA 2.0)

Top Actresses I Proclivities
Annex - Andrews, Julie_08 I https://www.flickr.com/photos/14141003@N05/9970308133/
Attribution 2.0 Generic (CC BY 2.0)

Top Actresses I Teresa Trimm
Audrey Hepburn colorized without added texture I https://www.flickr.com/photos/ttrimm/50829789871/
Attribution-ShareAlike 2.0 Generic (CC BY-SA 2.0)

Famous Icons I U.S. Embassy New Delhi
President John F. Kennedy I https://www.flickr.com/photos/usembassynewdelhi/5386861182/
Attribution-NoDerivs 2.0 Generic (CC BY-ND 2.0)

Famous Icons I Mike Licht
Martin Luther King, Jr. 1964 (source: Library of Congress) I https://www.flickr.com/photos/notionscapital/5360731135/
Attribution 2.0 Generic (CC BY 2.0)

Airliners I 1950sUnlimited
CAPITAL AIRLINES Viscount Powered By Rolls-Royce 60s I https://www.flickr.com/photos/blakta2/8268282684/
Attribution 2.0 Generic (CC BY 2.0)

Airliners I 1950sUnlimited
AMERICAN AIRLINES 707 Astrojet 60s I https://www.flickr.com/photos/blakta2/8267215735/
Attribution 2.0 Generic (CC BY 2.0)

Airliners I 1950sUnlimited
Saturn Airlines Douglas Super DC-8-61F jumbo airline issue postcard ca 1960s
https://www.flickr.com/photos/blakta2/8268275348/
Attribution 2.0 Generic (CC BY 2.0)

Vietnam War Photos I manhhai
Vietnam War 1960s - Navy Soldiers Walking with Bombers in Background
https://www.flickr.com/photos/13476480@N07/33931169848/
Attribution 2.0 Generic (CC BY 2.0)

Vietnam War Photos I manhhai
Vietnam War 1968 - Chris Noel I https://www.flickr.com/photos/13476480@N07/51443051661/
Attribution 2.0 Generic (CC BY 2.0)

Vietnam War Photos I manhhai
Vietnam War - VINH LONG INSTALLATION I https://www.flickr.com/photos/13476480@N07/51741102046/
Attribution 2.0 Generic (CC BY 2.0)

Kitchen Style I Ethan
https://www.flickr.com/photos/42353480@N02/5759547328/
Attribution 2.0 Generic (CC BY 2.0)

Kitchen Style I Ethan
1956 Hotpoint I https://www.flickr.com/photos/42353480@N02/5759004867/
Attribution 2.0 Generic (CC BY 2.0)

Kitchen Style I Ethan
https://www.flickr.com/photos/42353480@N02/5759001449/
Attribution 2.0 Generic (CC BY 2.0)

Women's Fashion I Ethan
NBH 1964 I https://www.flickr.com/photos/42353480@N02/8447193644/
Attribution 2.0 Generic (CC BY 2.0)

Women's Fashion I Ethan
NBH 1964 I https://www.flickr.com/photos/42353480@N02/8446107471/
Attribution 2.0 Generic (CC BY 2.0)

Women's Fashion I Ethan
NBH 1964 I https://www.flickr.com/photos/42353480@N02/8447193592/
Attribution 2.0 Generic (CC BY 2.0)

Living Room Decor I Ethan
1960 I https://www.flickr.com/photos/42353480@N02/6174536588
Attribution 2.0 Generic (CC BY 2.0)

Living Room Decor I Kevin
1960's Living Room I https://www.flickr.com/photos/kb35/4446267772/
Attribution 2.0 Generic (CC BY 2.0)

Living Room Decor I 1950sUnlimited
interior 1960s I https://www.flickr.com/photos/blakta2/8625062347
Attribution 2.0 Generic (CC BY 2.0)

Families I David Howard
family Highgate c1961 I https://www.flickr.com/photos/satguru/4589366822/
Attribution 2.0 Generic (CC BY 2.0)

Families I Joe Goldberg
Arthur and Mom I https://www.flickr.com/photos/goldberg/7539230/
Attribution-ShareAlike 2.0 Generic (CC BY-SA 2.0)

Families I Don O'Brien
1964 New York World's Fair I https://www.flickr.com/photos/dok1/4710345146/
Attribution 2.0 Generic (CC BY 2.0)

Famous Places I 1950sUnlimited
State Street Randolph, Chicago 64 I https://www.flickr.com/photos/blakta2/8542511927/
Attribution 2.0 Generic (CC BY 2.0)

Famous Places I 1950sUnlimited
miami beach florida 1964 I https://www.flickr.com/photos/blakta2/8268299608/
Attribution 2.0 Generic (CC BY 2.0)

Famous Places I 1950sUnlimited
Midway on Casino Pier & Rides - Seaside Park New Jersey
https://www.flickr.com/photos/blakta2/8268866802/
Attribution 2.0 Generic (CC BY 2.0)

Famous Places I Alex Dawson (theducks)
New York 2.jpg I https://www.flickr.com/photos/theducks/2267208322/
Attribution-ShareAlike 2.0 Generic (CC BY-SA 2.0)

Easter in the 60s I Don O'Brien
Christmas 1960 I https://www.flickr.com/photos/dok1/3133471314/
Attribution 2.0 Generic (CC BY 2.0)

Christmas in the 60s I Orange County Archives
Bud Hurlbut and family, Christmas 1960
https://www.flickr.com/photos/ocarchives/23906451017/
Attribution 2.0 Generic (CC BY 2.0)

Christmas in the 60s I alljengi
Christmas Day, Dec 1969
https://www.flickr.com/photos/27718315@N02/24641013694/
Attribution-ShareAlike 2.0 Generic (CC BY-SA 2.0)